THE MECHANICS
OF THE KNEE

HOW TO DEFEAT ARTHRITIS
AND IMPROVE MOBILITY
WITHOUT SURGERY

THE MECHANICS
OF THE KNEE

HOW TO DEFEAT ARTHRITIS
AND IMPROVE MOBILITY
WITHOUT SURGERY

DAVID C. MORLEY, JR., MD

NORTH LOOP BOOKS   MINNEAPOLIS, MN

North Loop Books
322 First Avenue N, 5th floor
Minneapolis, MN 55401
612.455.2294
www.NorthLoopBooks.com

ISBN-13: 978-1-63505-152-0
LCCN: PENDING

Distributed by Itasca Books

Cover Design by Emily Keenan
Typeset by C. Tramell

Printed in the United States of America

To my wife, Meg, who wrote the meaning of love into the pages of my heart.

CONTENTS

FOREWORD

"I can't walk today. My knee is killing me!" It's a complaint I hear all too often. In my thirty-five-year career as a family physician and sports clinician, I've had to assess and manage knee pain in athletes and especially in aging patients. Degenerative knee arthritis is the scourge of the baby boomers. In addition to the pain, restricted activity and secondary depression are the major challenges patients and health care providers face.

I have the good fortune of working closely with Dr. David Morley, Jr., an accomplished orthopedic surgeon. Over the years we have shared many patients suffering from knee arthritis. Many of these patients have successfully overcome their problems without resorting to surgery. The most gratifying results occur when patients "buy into the program." With weight loss, appropriate diet, and exercise, they can improve their functionality, pain, and outlook on life. Too often, orthopedic surgeons move directly to an operative approach. Many patients are desperate, since their quality of life has been eroded by their condition, and they want the quick results offered by surgery. Some do well, but many are left with a measure of discomfort.

Dr. Morley's book is a comprehensive and easy-reading guide to understanding and managing knee arthritis and the misery it can cause. He brings a career's worth of experience as a surgeon who has performed at the highest-quality level. This book is recommended for those who are at risk of knee arthritis, for current sufferers, and for family and friends who are supporting them.

Enjoy the read!

Mark Romanowsky, MD
Family Physician
UMASS Lowell Team Physician

ACKNOWLEDGMENTS

Over the years I have developed a great deal of affection for the people of the Pawtucket Falls area of the Merrimack Valley. I can say with great pride that "I have friends in Lowell places." It is no wonder that the unique, rough-and-tumble city of Lowell, Massachusetts, birthplace of the Industrial Revolution in North America, has produced such great writers, actors, and television hosts as Jack Kerouac, Bette Davis, and Ed McMahon. It has also brought us captains of industry like An Wang, Milton Bradley, and the Demoulas brothers. Famous politicians hail from Lowell, among them Paul Tsongas, Marty Meehan, and Mike Dukakis. But most of us are just regular folks. To paraphrase Saint Paul, who was not from Lowell, when he wrote to the Corinthians, the body is made up of many parts, all of which are essential. Each one of us contributes a little bit to the unfolding Lowell story. I wish to extend my thanks to the people of this miraculous community.

Special thanks go to my son, Anders, who showed great patience in editing and proofreading the manuscript of this book. If it is at all readable, he deserves the greater credit. Thanks are also owed to Dr. Mark Romanowsky, who watched as the book unfolded and made valuable comments that only he, as a seasoned primary-care physician, could make.

AUTHOR'S NOTE

This book is not a scientific treatise. Perhaps you will find it helpful and entertaining in an area that concerns your health. I can be very opinionated; ask anyone who knows me. The following pages contain many of my opinions and should not be used for self-treatment of knee arthritis. If you use it as such, you may need more than an orthopedic surgeon. You may need a psychiatrist. Sir William Osler, the legendary internist, famously said, "A physician who treats himself has a fool for a patient." A patient who acts as his own physician is even worse off. So if you have an orthopedic problem, consult your primary-care physician, who may send you to an orthopedist.

This book is meant to help educate readers concerning the small world of adult reconstructive orthopedic surgery, in which I've lived for the last three decades. It is said that the truth will set you free. I've tried to capture my treatment methodology for knee arthritis. The approach found here is based on my medical education, my life "on the streets" of Lowell, thirty years as an active and board-certified orthopedic surgeon in private practice, and exhaustive reading and study in the area of knee arthritis. It is my hope that applying the principles in this book will set you free from the pain associated with this disease.

But always bear in mind that opinions will vary, even among experts. Very little of what I suggest is controversial, but where there is disagreement I have done my best to make that clear. Contrary to what some surgeons might suggest, I do not believe arthritis can be "cured." So if you're looking for a magic remedy to the complex problem of knee arthritis, this book is not for you. In my experience, damage to the articular cartilage in your knee is permanent. What we can do, however, is control and even minimize symptoms using a structured program that may well make surgery unnecessary. In some cases, the worsening of arthritis can be decreased. As Benjamin Franklin said, "An ounce of prevention is worth a pound of cure."

INTRODUCTION

While on sabbatical recently, I had the enjoyable experience of studying Ancient Greek. I applied my newly acquired ability during a tour of both Greece and Turkey (Asia Minor, to Greek scholars), where I could translate some of the ancient writings found in and around Athens, Corinth, Ephesus, and Troy. It was a once-in-a-lifetime experience. Through it I learned that many English words are based on Greek roots. For example, the word osteoarthritis comes from the Greek *osteo*, meaning "bone"; *arthro*, meaning "joint"; and *itis*, meaning "inflammation." Quite literally, then, osteoarthritis is inflammation of the bone and joint. In fact, osteoarthritis (OA) is more accurately designated osteoarthrosis, since there may be minimal inflammation associated with the condition. Nevertheless, although perhaps not etymologically correct, throughout this book I will refer to osteoarthritis as simply arthritis or OA.

Ideally, a physician should be both a healer and teacher. Patients need to be taught about arthritis of the knee. Evidence shows that the incidence of knee osteoarthritis has increased in our society. The probability of developing this disease by the age of eighty-five is approximately 50 percent. For the past thirty years I have practiced orthopedic surgery in Lowell, Massachusetts. In that time I have witnessed a dramatic rise in the number of knee arthritis cases. In my office I see a complete spectrum of this disease, from the mild, aching discomfort consistent with early arthritis to full-blown late-stage arthritis, characterized by swelling, stiffness, loss of motion, and marked pain made worse by walking in the presence of bone-on-bone changes visible on x-rays. This book is restricted primarily to a discussion of what is commonly known as osteoarthritis, degenerative joint disease, or wear-and-tear arthritis of the knee.

Some would say that we see more knee arthritis today because, thanks to medical advances, people live longer, and the condition is a disease of old age. There may be some truth to this. In 1900 the average person lived to be about forty-six. By 1950 the average life expectancy had increased to around sixty-five. Today, a healthy baby can expect to live for more than eighty years. With age comes infirmity, including arthritis.

In the first section of *The Mechanics of the Knee*, we will look at the complex design and workings of the normal knee. We will then examine what changes occur to the normal knee, resulting in arthritis. In the second section, armed with a solid understanding of the problem, we can implement the treatment of this disabling condition on several fronts—applied mechanics, physical therapy, and medications—thus taking back our mobility. Once we have achieved mastery over the disease, in the third section we will learn how to stop the progression of arthritis through correct lifestyle choices.

Contrary to what some suggest, I do not believe that arthritis is a "natural" disease. Many joints age without progressive degenerative changes occurring. Although arthritis may be seen more commonly in the elderly than the young, it is not the result of a progressive deterioration as a result of age. The knee is a very complex and vulnerable joint. There is, granted, in some families a hereditary predisposition to develop arthritis in certain joints. But while overuse—particularly repetitive heavy-impact loading and obesity— can cause damage to the articular cartilage, normal vigorous activity has the reverse effect: the cartilage can actually become *healthier*. Exercise can benefit those with established arthritis by relieving inflammation, restoring motion, and improving muscle tone and girth. The challenge, in my opinion, is not to find out how long we can extend a hollow, nonproductive life filled with aches and pains but to extend a vigorous, relatively pain-free, productive life full of meaning and unimpeded by the shackles of OA.

We live in a postindustrial digital age. We have secured the blessings of mechanization and computers but also their curses. The quantity and the variety of the food we eat in this country have never been greater as a result of science. Food is not only conveniently available but also quickly prepared and often processed. This synthetic food is, in many cases, filled with more calories (and less taste) than the real food slowly prepared by our ancestors. Along with scientifically altered food come a multitude of preservatives and stabilizing chemicals. This toxic cornucopia can be reviewed on the nutritional label of any can or package containing processed "food." Additives also include sugar, salt, fat, and high-fructose corn syrup—all of which have negative health effects.

Moreover, as the margins between day and night have become blurred, many of us retire late at night and sleep in, disrupting our natural circadian rhythms. Meals are eaten erratically, in large portions, and consist of the wrong types of food—all resulting in weight gain. It is not unusual for people to have a large doughnut with coffee for breakfast and then to snack throughout the day on food packed with sugar and fat, only to return home famished. In a feeding frenzy, they eat enormous amounts of food of the wrong kind. After collapsing in an exhausted stupor to hypnotically watch reality TV, they wake up after the eleven o'clock news, starving for a midnight snack. They may pop a sleeping pill before turning in for a restless six hours of sleep, then wake up exhausted to repeat the whole sequence of events. This dangerous cycle leads to a slow process of weight gain and breakdown—both physical and mental.

In the words of Henry David Thoreau, we need to "simplify." When I was a child in Kingston, Ontario, I would walk one mile to school and back in all seasons. (I admit, I did not walk uphill in both directions like my grandpa did.) Since we were relatively poor, breakfast consisted of old-fashioned oatmeal with powdered milk, topped with a small amount of brown sugar. Our family did not own a car until I was six years old. We walked everywhere. Prior to the 1950s, most people walked far more than we do in the twenty-first century. In the old days it was not unusual for a normal, healthy person to walk ten miles daily. Looking through old books about life in New England, I have found accounts of people who routinely walked up to 120 miles a week. And the distance was often covered on rough roads or paths.

This stands in stark contrast to today's elementary-grade students who are driven from their houses to the end of the driveway to wait for the school bus. Is it any wonder that there is an epidemic of obesity in our young people? A rough rule of thumb is that a person walking one mile burns approximately seventy calories. In *On the Road*, Jack Kerouac (our most famous native son here in Lowell) wrote, "Whither goest thou, America, in thy shiny car in the night?" The car has been both a blessing and curse. It has freed us to go places we could not previously go and to enjoy fuller lives. It has enabled us, in many cases, to live suburban lifestyles surrounded by stuff (accompanied by long commutes to work). From a physical-health perspective, cars have been a disaster, translating to people exercising less and burning fewer calories every day. From a psychological point of view, being trapped in a car for hours may lead to a feeling of social isolation and loss of community, which may blossom into deep-seated anger and depression. This explains the phenomenon of road rage. You can see the results of such disconnectedness all around you as the seeds of despair sprout—broken families, disappearing community and religious values, drug and alcohol addiction, and, of course, arthritic knees.

How do we emerge from this dangerous downward spiral? Get back to basics. Walk. Ride your bike. Swim. Ski. Move! And eat good food. Love people. Take time to smell the roses.

In 2011 I visited the central hospital in Bergamo, Italy, and had the delight of touring the orthopedic facilities with the orthopedic surgeon-in-chief. I was surprised that in this northern Italian hospital, the incidence of knee replacement was approximately one quarter of what I had observed in Lowell. In general, I noticed that the citizens of Bergamo, a very hilly region, walked virtually everywhere. In addition, the food was uniformly made the old-fashioned way (from scratch) and was healthy. It was prepared from fresh, naturally grown ingredients, flavored with spices and extra-virgin olive oil, and was enjoyed with wine in moderation.

As a result of our society's "devolution," we've developed many degenerative diseases, including arthritis of the knee. In this book I will explore why the incidence of knee arthritis has risen so drastically and offer my expert advice on how we can reverse the trend. Prior to the 1960s, there were few options for the treatment of knee arthritis. The doctor might recommend aspirin for control of pain and a cane to help with walking. The modern era of knee arthritis treatment did not begin in earnest until the early 1970s. As the incidence of knee arthritis has increased, we've seen a dramatic growth in the number of surgeries done on the knee—especially total knee replacement (arthroplasty). This operation, which used to be reserved for end-stage arthritis, is now done routinely for the treatment of moderately advanced arthritis, often without first exhausting conservative measures. Unquestionably, there is a place for total knee replacement—but only as a last resort. One of my colleagues has described knee replacement as a salvage operation for bone-on-bone arthritis.

In my opinion, many patients make the decision to proceed with total replacement prematurely. This book has been written as an encouragement to patients to continue the good fight using conservative measures and try to avoid throwing in the towel before they are *really* ready for knee arthroplasty.

Dr. Lanny Johnson, an internationally famous arthroscopic surgeon, has characterized knee replacement as "internal amputation." Although this statement is dramatic, it gets the point across. Once a biological joint is removed and replaced with plastic and metal, an irreversible step has been taken. Furthermore, joint replacement, although it often yields an acceptable result, seldom yields a great one. Many patients experience a marginal outcome with continued problems, such as achiness, numbness, swelling, stiffness, and loss of function that often require the use of a cane and occasionally a knee brace. The resolute and reasoned patient waits until the proper time—after conservative measures have failed.

When I initially went into private practice I joined a senior orthopedist by the name of Howard Harrison. This experienced physician and surgeon taught me a great deal about people and disease. One day he called me into an examining room. Before me, I saw an older gentleman in his early eighties. Dr. Harrison explained to me that this man had been a paratrooper during World War II and had made a jump in Normandy on D-Day. I looked at the patient with great respect. He was a healthy, spry, dignified man, who appeared sinewy yet strong. He had "bowed" legs as though he were a cowboy who had just gotten off his horse. On observation, he was noted to have good muscle tone and girth in the thigh and calf muscles. When he moved his knees, crunching was audible, but he made no complaints of pain. Despite the bowing of his knees, they were not unstable. Moreover, he had only mild discomfort when I pressed on the joint lines. I could feel the ridges of bone spurs present but caused him no pain when I touched them. There was no heat, redness, or swelling when I examined his knees, and his motion was almost full.

But then Dr. Harrison showed me the x-rays of his knees—severe bone-on-bone arthritis. Based on a review of the horrible x-ray appearance of his knees, I concluded that he would benefit from total knee replacements. But he denied knee pain! I was confused. The senior physician finally took pity and explained to me that the patient was at the office for evaluation of his right elbow. It seems that the man could only play two to three sets of tennis without elbow pain. I looked at the radiographs again. Had these two rascals switched x-rays on me? Impossible. The physical alignment of his knees matched the x-ray appearance. What was going on? Dr. Harrison laughed and asked, "Did you just learn something?" Indeed I had. Before me was a recon paratrooper, apparently bulletproof and invincible. I had known some of these guys at Camp Pendleton in California. They were a breed apart. The patient confirmed this as he looked at me with a twinkle in his eye. So what was his secret? He controlled his weight and continued to lead an active lifestyle in advanced age. I could see his curiosity and fun-loving nature as he played a good joke on the "young doc." I returned home later that day and said to my wife, "You won't believe this guy I met in the office today!"

In 1970 and 1971 I had the privilege of serving in the United States Marine Corps. While at Parris Island, South Carolina, I was taught the meaning of integrity and endurance. I encourage my patients to show those same attributes, which have made America great and have guaranteed our freedom. May your fight against arthritis free you from joint pain and disability.

Semper fi.

PART ONE

UNDERSTANDING THE KNEE AND KNEE ARTHRITIS

CHAPTER 1

THE KNEE IN HEALTH

What is arthritis of the knee? Who does it affect? What is its incidence and impact on society? Who is at risk, and what factors predispose some people to its development? Can the onset and progression of knee arthritis be avoided or minimized? Are there stages of severity? What can I do to avoid it, and how can I treat it when it occurs?

Before we can adequately address these questions, we need to learn more about the knee in health. In this chapter we will take a look at the parts of the knee and how they work together as a functional system (the anatomy and mechanics of the knee). Once these building blocks have been laid, we will understand what normal is and will be in a position to evaluate the abnormal knee. The abnormal, or diseased, knee will be the subject of the second chapter. And in chapter three we will look at how doctors examine the knee and assess its condition using clinical studies like x-rays and MRIs.

BONES—THE SUPPORTING SUPERSTRUCTURE

Bones are the girders on which the soft tissue of your body depends for strength and anchoring. Like the I-beam steel in skyscrapers, bones are very strong. They are made of both organic material (soft tissue such as collagen) and inorganic material (minerals like calcium and phosphorus). The calcium and phosphorus are infused within a matrix of soft tissue that provides tremendous strength. We can imagine them as bricks in mortar. But unlike a brick wall, bone is a living material and changes throughout our lives. Young bones contain more cartilage than old. That's why children seem to bend when they fall, like Gumby, without breaking. Have you ever tried to snap a green willow stick, only to have it crack on one side but not the other? The same thing can happen to children when long bones like the arm or shinbones fracture. A greenstick break may lead to the unfortunate circumstance of the orthopedic surgeon having to "complete the fracture." Only a clean break enables straightening before a plaster cast or splint can be applied to set the bone properly.

Unlike kids, however, adults don't bend. They fracture sometimes after minimal trauma. Sedentary lifestyle, improper diet, or simply increasing age can result in a gradual leaching of the calcium and phosphorus (the bricks) from the bone, resulting in a decrease of mechanical strength. The mineral loss is also brought about by hormonal changes in our bodies. Postmenopausal women experience a deficiency in estrogen that leads to osteopenia (thinning of the bones) or osteoporosis (porosity of the bones). Both conditions result in progressive loss of bone strength. All of these factors contribute to the increased fragility of our bones as we grow older. In more severe forms, a fracture of insufficiency may occur, when even mild trauma may result in a broken bone. It is therefore important to eat foods with adequate amounts of calcium and phosphorus so the body can maintain the strength of the bone. In addition, it is important to get adequate amounts of vitamin D (the sunshine vitamin) and exercise, which we will discuss in chapter six.

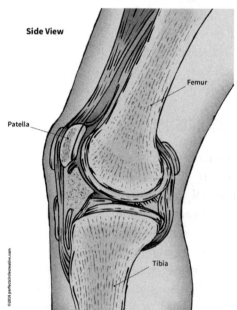

Diagram 1

Two bones that are very important for understanding the knee are the femur and tibia (see diagram 1).

Both are long bones with hollow shafts, like golf clubs. The thick walls of the shafts are called the cortex and comprise the strong and resilient composite of organic tissue and minerals we touched on above. Toward the end of the femur and at the upper portion of the tibia, the space between the thick walls is filled with cancellous, or spongy, bone. This porous bone distributes stress from within the knee joint into the shaft of the bone, acting as a shock absorber.

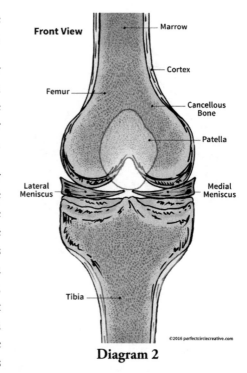

Diagram 2

The study of anatomy—our physical structure—uses its own special language to describe the parts of the body and their interrelationships (see diagram 2).

The knee is the joint, or articulation, between the femur (thigh bone) and the tibia (shin bone). Aspect is the technical term that describes the perspective from which you look at something. In anatomy, the inner aspect of the knee joint (where the perspective is from between your legs) is called the medial aspect. The outer side is known as the lateral aspect. The back is posterior, while the front is anterior. In addition to the femur and the tibia, there is a third bone in the anterior part of the knee. It is called the patella, or kneecap, and belongs to a special group of bones called sesamoids—bones that are embedded in tendons (rather than being hinged to each other, like the femur and tibia).

Anatomy also has words to describe the complex movements that the three joints of the knee make. When we straighten the knee, it is called extension, while when we bend it, we speak of flexion. The knee is also capable of rotation (pivoting) and translation (sliding back and forth). I like to describe these motions as bending and rolling, spinning, and gliding and sliding.

What we call the knee joint actually consists of three separate joints, which we sometimes call compartments (see diagrams 1 and 2). The joints on either side of the knee are known as the medial and lateral compartments, while the joint at the front and center of the knee is called the patella-femoral compartment (because it describes the articulation between the patella and the front of the femur). The patella glides in an anterior femoral groove as

Cross Section

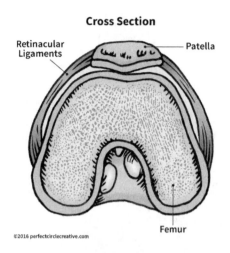

Retinacular Ligaments

Patella

Femur

©2016 perfectcirclecreative.com

Diagram 3

we bend our knees, in much the same way as a monorail train glides along its single track (see diagram 3).

Occasionally, the ligaments (which we will discuss in a few pages) that stabilize the inner and outer aspect of the patella to the femur will be torn, and the train will jump the track, resulting in a patellar dislocation. The patella is inserted into the quadriceps and patellar tendons and acts, in mechanical terms, as a fulcrum. By raising the tendons (which work together as a contractible lever) away from the femur, the patella enhances the leverage of the knee, thereby increasing extension force by a factor of two. As a consequence, patients who have their patellas removed will lose half of the straightening power of the knee. This becomes a real problem when trying to climb stairs (which is why removal of the kneecap—and the resultant debilitation—is a last resort for surgeons but a favorite punishment of mafia dons).

A second compartment of the knee joint involves the medial aspect (i.e., the right side of the left knee and the left side of the right knee). This movement takes place in the articulation between the medial femoral condyle (each of the familiar knobs at the lower extremity of the femur) and the medial part of the tibia. The condyle acts as a roller, rotating and pivoting on the upper portion of the tibia, in a very complex motion that is guided by the ligaments. Finally, the lateral compartment is home to the coordinated movement between the lateral femoral condyle and the upper outer aspect of the tibia. The three parts of the knee are always working as a complex ensemble, never as soloists, keeping orthopedic surgeons on their toes!

Another important consideration is the alignment of the femur with respect to the tibia. A valgus aligned knee is a condition in which the knee joint is bent into the centerline of the body. This is called being "knock-kneed" (see diagram 4).

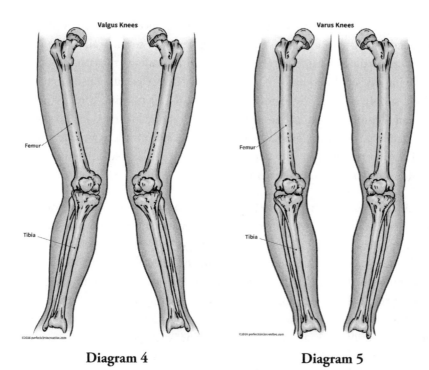

Diagram 4   **Diagram 5**

On the other hand, being "bow-legged" suggests that the knee is bent out from the centerline of the body (see diagram 5).

People with marked alignment abnormalities are often prone to developing arthritis because of the abnormal stresses that occur on the knee joint.

CARTILAGE—THE RUBBER ON THE KNEE-TIRE

Lining the lower part of the femur, the upper part of the tibia, and the back of the patella is a miraculous coating called hyaline, or articular, cartilage. The word hyaline comes from a Greek word that means glasslike. As the name suggests, it has a bluish-pink smooth and glassy surface. The texture of hyaline cartilage is like the rubber tread of your car tire. The area of the bone to which the cartilage adheres is called the subchondral bone. Hyaline cartilage's Teflon-like surface is five times as slippery as ice. It is about a quarter-inch thick and quite durable. I've seen many ninety-year-olds whose hyaline cartilage has still not worn out—that's a lot of miles! This magical lining is made up of several layers, and its surface may delaminate after injuries. In some cases, the cartilage fragments float around, enlarging with time, and become stuck within the knee. Orthopedic surgeons call these fragments "joint mice" because of their tendency to sneak around the joint. They can result in a catching sensation noted by patients that causes locking or giving out of the joint. If it wears away or is peeled off, cartilage has no blood supply and cannot regrow, leaving the femur to grind directly on the tibia in a condition sometimes called bone-on-bone arthritis. It also has no nerve supply. But that's probably a good thing, since if there were sensation, we'd feel every bump in the road as a painful shock in our knees. Running would hurt worse than it already does.

If you looked at hyaline cartilage under the microscope and analyzed it biochemically, you would see that it is made up of four components: water, proteoglycans, collagen, and cartilage cells. At 80 percent of the total makeup, water is the most abundant of these four elements. But the remaining 20 percent has a lot of good stuff in it. As their name suggests, proteoglycans (PGs) are made up of protein and sugar. They are miraculous structures that call to mind those little clear pearls in tapioca pudding. On closer inspection with an electron microscope, each pearl looks like a mini-hairbrush with many bristles. They act like sponges; if water is squeezed out, it can be rapidly reabsorbed. When weight is applied to cartilage, the PGs contained within it bend, mold, and twist, but once the pressure is removed they miraculously snap back to their original shape—just like a good coif. The collagen component is the glue, or the pudding, if you will, that holds all the tapioca pearls together. Now, I know what you're asking yourself: "What is the matrix?" Okay, maybe that's just what I was asking myself. The matrix—Neo could have asked me and avoided a lot of trouble—is the combination of collagen and proteoglycans. Sprinkled through the water and matrix pudding are tiny cells, chondrocytes (cartilage cells), which produce new matrix as needed.

Like any surface, cartilage can be broken down. It can be damaged suddenly, as a result of direct impact during trauma, or it can be slowly worn away. Wear and tear may occur over time as a result of an increased load being applied for a prolonged period. Obesity has been identified as one such cause of consumption. Just as if you were to overload an old Ford pickup truck with bags of cement and then drive down a pot-holed country road, you'll destroy the shocks and eventually crack the frame. Sudden damage to the cartilage can occur during collision sports, such as football, which not only repeatedly overload the bearing surface—through hard running and pivoting—but also often injure the lining of the knee by direct impact. Mechanical stresses, like thumping and bumping around instead of walking gracefully, or carrying heavy objects on a regular or recurrent basis, can also lead to progressive cartilage destruction and eventually arthritis. This is why physicians see higher rates of knee arthritis in workers whose jobs involve heavy and prolonged weight-bearing activities, like bending, kneeling, squatting, lifting, stair and ladder climbing, and carrying heavy loads. The problem is common enough that some doctors classify osteoarthritis as a weight-bearing disease.

Unfortunately, not all cartilage is created equal. Poor-quality bearing cartilage can be inherited genetically. Blame your parents if you don't have designer "treads." Suffice it to say that good cartilage lasts longer than bad. It has been my observation that knee arthritis simply runs in some families.

There is another type of cartilage called meniscal cartilage (see diagram 6).

Top View

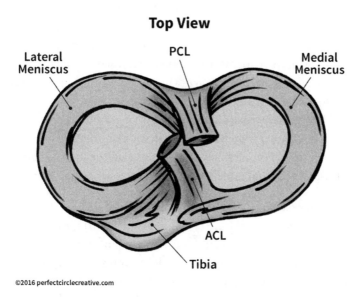

Lateral Meniscus

PCL

Medial Meniscus

ACL

Tibia

©2016 perfectcirclecreative.com

Diagram 6

Confusion occurs because doctors refer to it as a meniscus, while lay people call it a cartilage. The menisci are two cartilage gaskets that act like cushions between the bottom of the femur and top of the tibia. When people say, "I tore my cartilage," they mean they have ripped one of their menisci.

Meniscus comes originally from a Greek word that means little or crescent moon. The two cartilages in your knee are shaped like crescent moons, or parentheses, that face inward toward each other from either side of the joint (diagram 6). The menisci have three basic functions. First, they are shock absorbers and protect healthy hyaline cartilage. If these spacers are removed, the joint load between the femur and the tibia increases by 100 percent, resulting in a gradual wearing away of the hyaline cartilage. The second function of the menisci is to fill the gap between the rounded ends of the femur and tibia, acting as stabilizers and shims. If they are torn or removed surgically, the knee may become loose or unstable. The resulting condition is called a "trick knee." Thirdly, the menisci serve a lubricating purpose, wetting down the hyaline cartilage of the femur, tibia, and patella with joint fluid and thus maintaining a healthy and clean bearing surface.

SYNOVIUM—THE INNER LINING

A semi-waterproof sheet, acting as a casing for the synovial fluid (SF), lines the knee joint internally. Known as the synovium, this pink membrane is a specialized pliable overlay similar to the layer that protects the cornea of your eyes. Many of my patients, on viewing arthroscopic images of the knee, tell me it looks like seaweed. The synovium produces a slippery liquid—the synovial fluid—that sustains and lubricates the cartilage. Just like the lining of the eye that produces tears when irritated by an onion, when the synovium is insulted (for example, when the knee is injured or inflamed) it responds by producing excessive SF, sometimes called "water on the knee." Normally, less than one teaspoon of fluid circulates in the knee joint, acting like Slick 50.

A very important part of the synovial fluid is hyaluronic acid (HA). HA traps water molecules, and the resulting HA-water composite lubricates the hyaline cartilage surface, creating almost friction-free motion of the joint. In arthritis, less HA is produced, resulting in poor lubrication and increased friction within the knee. Articular cartilage injury during weight-bearing stress, like walking or running, may result. Like properly greased ball bearings, well-lubricated hyaline cartilage decreases friction. Worn or broken ball bearings lead to overheating, noise, vibration, difficulty turning, locking up, and the eventual need for replacement. Anyone who has ever seen a trailer wheel with malfunctioning ball bearings knows the scenario: the wheel heats up, starts to smoke as it turns bright red, and eventually seizes. This is often accompanied by a screeching noise and the explosion of the tire. Although not as spectacular in the human knee, the result may be the same—immobility. As we will discuss later, synthetic HA preparations (viscosupplementation) have been introduced to replace the hyaluronic acid lost in arthritis.

Often inflammation or trauma can produce increased fluid in the knee. If distended, the knee begins to hurt. Like an overfilled water balloon, it becomes tense and unbending. Some of my most grateful patients have been those who have simply had their knees drained. Moreover, certain conditions, such as autoimmune diseases like rheumatoid arthritis and lupus, affect the synovium. Such cases are classified as inflammatory arthritis. When the synovium becomes sick, it may produce SF of poor quality or insufficient quantity. The articular cartilage often soon degrades. Osteoarthritis, on the other hand, affects primarily the articular cartilage and not the synovium.

LIGAMENTS—THE GUY WIRES HOLDING THINGS TOGETHER

In anatomical terms, ligaments are fibrous connective tissue that attaches one bone to another. Complex networks of ligaments are found around and inside the knee and are the primary stabilizers of the joint. Picture a ligament as woven manila rope. The cord is made of many hemp fibers. I think of ligaments as being high-tech ropes filled with electronic sensors that tell your joints how much force is being applied to them. The e-sensors, or nerve receptors, are attached to nerve fibers within the ligaments that line your knee. These delicate nerves tell your brain the position of the knee joint. Is it straight or bent? We call this proprioception, or your awareness of joint placement. If a ligament is torn or injured, this very important proprioceptive function may be destroyed.

Ligaments are static (not moving) and designed to allow no stretch. They hold joints together and permit a limited number of motions to occur. Although it's tempting to think of the knee as a simple hinge joint, it's far more complicated. It not only flexes and extends but also rotates and slightly translates (shifts from front to back). Elvis could also gyrate—a signature pelvic move that the King perfected. The collateral ligaments, which are on the inside and outside of the knee, guide it through flexion and extension while preventing side-to-side bending. At the expense of motion comes stability. Without the collateral ligaments, our knees would collapse.

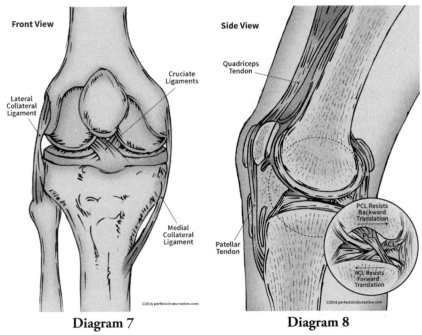

Diagram 7   **Diagram 8**

Another set of ligaments controls the complex rotational and translational motion of the knee. These are the cruciate ligaments (see diagram 7).

The anterior and posterior cruciate ligaments (ACL and PCL) cross one another inside the knee (cruciate means cross-shaped). Sometimes people call them the "crucial ligaments" because they are important stabilizers of the knee during pivoting-type motions. Think of a halfback suddenly cutting to avoid being tackled. The player is able to do this because of the stabilizing effect of the ACL. Without the ligament his knee would "spin out," and he would fall flat on the ground. The ACL is found in the center of the knee and passes from the inside front of the tibia (shin bone) to the back and outer portion of the femur (thigh bone) (see diagram 8).

It is wrapped in a sheath of synovium and is composed of three large bundles of ligament fibers. Within the ligament are nerves and stretch receptors. Unfortunately, when the ACL is torn, proprioceptive function is lost. A similar situation results when the PCL is torn. Since the PCL is twice as strong as the ACL, however, it is seldom ripped completely. The anterior cruciate ligament prevents the forward motion of the tibia on the femur, while the stronger posterior crucial ligament prevents the backward motion of the tibia on the femur.

The ACL is often injured during trauma that causes excessive twisting of the knee. That is why a "clipping injury" in football carries such a large penalty. It can result in the requirement for surgery and can be a career ender. Even though surgeons have become quite skilled at reconstructing a torn ACL, and stability may be achieved, they cannot rebuild the nerves within the ligament, and proprioception is never restored. This may be one reason why even reconstructed knees eventually often develop arthritis.

The patella too is guided in its complex course along the end of the femur by the retinacular ligaments, which restrain its side-to-side excursion, much like guy wires (diagram 3). These broad, thin ligaments of the knee guide the femur, tibia, and patella through a complex motion determined by their unique architecture. When the ligaments of the knee are torn, abnormal motion can result, often leading to arthritis. Physicians call this "secondary arthritis" because it occurs as a late result of trauma. We refer to garden-variety arthritis, which occurs with aging and wear and tear, as osteoarthritis or primary arthritis.

MUSCLES—THE TURBO-CHARGED MOTORS

The knee joint is surrounded by some of the strongest muscles in the body. These "kick-butt" muscles propel us through life. In the front part of the thigh are the quadriceps muscles. In the back part are the hamstring muscles. Muscles attach to bones by way of tendons, or cords. Think of the muscle as a motor and a tendon as a cable. Just like a motorized winch pulls on its cable, a muscle, when it contracts, pulls on its tendon, causing the joint to move. So in the front of the knee we have the quadriceps muscle, attached by means of the quadriceps tendon to the patella, which in turn is joined by the patellar tendon to the upper tibia. As we discussed, the patella gives a mechanical advantage to the knee by effectively doubling the force of extension; in other words, this little bone enables the quadriceps muscle to do more with the same amount of energy. Now that's teamwork.

Although we normally think of the muscles of the thigh in terms of motors that help us move around, they have two other very important functions: acting as shock absorbers and dynamic (moving) stabilizers. Muscles decrease shock by damping out the bumps in the road. The damaging effect of repetitive impact loading on normal, healthy articular cartilage is well accepted medically. In the presence of quadriceps weakness, the impact passing up the leg to the knee, generated while walking, can be many times your body weight when your heel hits the ground. Wow! That's a lot of force. That's why Dr. Morley says, "Keep your weight down, your legs strong, and walk like a ninja." One medical guru stated that the amount of energy produced during normal walking would be enough to tear the ligaments of your legs apart if it were not for the muscles absorbing the shock. But you intuitively know this to be true. Did you ever step off a curb not knowing there was a drop? The jar that comes rattles your rafters from the belfry to the cellar. President Bill Clinton tore his quadriceps completely while descending a step unexpectedly and required surgical repair. These unexpected sudden loads are thought to be a contributing cause of wear-and-tear arthritis. Muscle weakness and nerve damage (peripheral neuropathy), which may occur as a result of aging, diabetes, vitamin deficiencies, or other factors, will decrease your leg muscles' ability to act as effective shock absorbers. Add to this poor balance, and the result may be someone who literally crashes through life. You've heard them: thump, thump, thump—crash. As they careen, thump, bump, and trip their way down life's road, they may be damaging their articular cartilage at each step, leading to progressive arthritic changes. Have you ever seen an exhausted, dehydrated Boston Marathoner descending the hill from Boston College? Some of these athletes are so used up that their feet slap the ground, reflecting extreme leg muscle fatigue and weakness as they painfully trudge on. They're not doing their cartilage and bone any favors. Their joints are being exposed to the full ground reaction force without any protective muscle shock absorption. I can remember, as a resident at the Roosevelt Hospital in New York City, taking care of an overweight middle-aged marathoner who, at the eighth mile of the New York Marathon, noted sudden pain in his groin and shortening of his leg. As a result of muscle weakness, extra weight, and repetitive impact loading, he sustained a stress fracture through the neck of his femur that completely displaced in a very dramatic and unexpected fashion. For this wounded athlete, surgery was the only reasonable option.

Along with the primary static ligament stabilizers, muscles can act as secondary dynamic stabilizers, changing tension on the basis of contraction. If, for example, your knee suddenly gives out, the quadriceps and hamstring muscles may reflexively contract to keep you from falling. The hamstring muscles dynamically stabilize the knee, similar to the way the ACL does. The quadriceps muscles dynamically give support to the knee like the PCL.

BURSAS—THE AIRBAGS

Bursas are little protective sacs found throughout the body, particularly around the knee. They pad the underlying bones, muscles, and tendons. Normally they're collapsed on themselves, but they can rapidly fill with fluid after direct injury. They can become hot and red when infected—a condition called septic bursitis—and require antibiotics and sometimes drainage. The biggest bursa in the knee, found in front of the kneecap, is called the pre-patellar bursa. Because the bursas protect tendons, they can be inflamed along with the underlying tendons. That's why doctors often see tendinitis and bursitis together. In many cases, it's difficult to determine whether the pain is coming from tendinitis or bursitis. In general, bursas are not involved in osteoarthritis.

THE PHYSICS OF THE KNEE—HOW IT WORKS

The articulation or joining of the femur, tibia, and patella is complicated, as we have seen. The science that studies the structure and function of the knee is called biomechanics. In order to understand the causes and treatment of arthritis, we should understand some basics.

The term biomechanics comes from ancient Greek and means "the mechanics of life." This branch of physics studies analytically all the parts and functions of the knee—bone, cartilage, tendons, ligaments, muscles—and their interactions, both with each other and with their environment. As in other branches of physics, practical engineering principles can be applied to the study of the knee. Bioengineers study not only the materials of the knee but the motion and forces, both normal and abnormal, acting on the joint. The forces that occur on the knee are very significant and change with activities. For example, being overweight results in increased stress on the joint, even when performing light activities, such as standing and walking. Excessive impact-loading type activities, such as stomping, running, and jumping, can result in injury to the knee over a period of time. Once joint damage has occurred, as in arthritis, impact loading aggravates or accelerates the deterioration of the knee joint. Stair climbing increases the patella-femoral joint load up to four times body weight and sometimes even more. A two-hundred-pound man generates eight hundred pounds of pressure across the patella-femoral joint. Standing from a squatted position markedly increases the load on articular cartilage. Jumping up from a crouched position may place pressures across the kneecap of over ten times body weight. It's not surprising that competitive weight lifters ascending from a squat can rip their patellar tendons off the bone in a dramatic fashion as a result of the incredible stress placed across the knee.

An important concept for understanding biomechanics is ground reaction force (GRF). The GRF is the force applied to a body by the ground. In other words, when you stand on the ground, the ground pushes back at you. It reminds me of Chuck Norris; when I do a push-up, I push myself away from the ground, but when Chuck Norris does one, he pushes the earth away from him. Very simply, when you stand, the ground reaction force is your body weight—the effect of gravity. If you lived on the moon, you would weigh one-sixth of what you do on Earth. As a 150-pound man, I would weigh twenty-five pounds. I could be an Olympic long jumper and win! But alas, even though your spouse might think it's a great idea, being sent to the moon is not a viable treatment for arthritis. During normal walking, a force load occurs across the knee joint of almost five times body weight. If you gain ten pounds, you're placing fifty pounds more force across your knee joint at each step! Other investigators have shown that each pound of weight you lose represents a four-pound reduction in knee joint load. Now you can understand why losing weight is so important to the health of your knee.

In addition to force, biomechanics also studies knee motion. When your knee is out straight, we call that zero degrees. When you are sitting in a chair with your foot flat on the floor, your knee is usually at around 90 degrees. The normal knee flexion is approximately zero to 140 degrees. Everyday activities, like walking, stair climbing, and getting up out of a chair, require around zero to 120 degrees. Arthritic bone spurs (bone projections along the joint line) growing within the knee that act as mechanical blocks to movement can decrease knee motion. Disruption of the joint surface alters the proper bending of the knee and can result in stiffness and motion loss. Too much fat under the skin at the back of the knee prevents flexion. This is another reason it is so important for those with knee arthritis to work on flexibility and weight loss. Increased motion leads to better movement.

Knowledge is power. We can now begin to apply our knowledge of the anatomy and the biomechanics of the knee to an understanding of knee arthritis. In the next two chapters we'll take a look at the symptoms and signs of knee arthritis and the tools used by orthopedists to analyze it, before moving on to part two of the book, where we will look at possibilities for treatment.

CHAPTER 2

ARTHRITIS OF THE KNEE

Before we learn how to free ourselves from the constraints of knee arthritis, we must understand the disease that is holding us back. In the first chapter we laid the foundation for this understanding with an overview of the anatomy of the knee and a few relevant aspects of biomechanics. In this chapter, I want to define some basic building blocks of osteoarthritis. The blocks I am going to consider are the signs and symptoms of arthritis, its causes, its outlook, its impact on lifestyle, and finally a brief look at other diseases that affect the knee.

KNEE OSTEOARTHRITIS—A DEGENERATIVE DISEASE

I mentioned in the introduction that the word osteoarthritis (OA) stems from three Greek roots meaning bone, joint, and inflammation. Osteoarthritis is most commonly described as a disease characterized by inflammation of the joints (which, as we saw in chapter one, are made of bones, cartilage, and many other parts). This is a handy but overly simple definition; that's because, as I also said in the introduction, in some cases there may be little or no inflammation—which is why we have another term, osteoarthrosis, that is sometimes used by those who insist on hair-splitting linguistic accuracy. Also, the term arthritis is used to describe some one hundred different diseases whose common feature is joint inflammation.

OA is the most common of the many types of arthritis, and it is the variety I am focusing on in this book. It can be characterized as a degenerative disease, and in fact is often called degenerative arthritis or simply degenerative joint disease. A degenerative disease is one that progressively worsens with time—

that is, unless something is done to slow down the process of degeneration. Although it occurs in many joints, we are interested in OA as it affects your knees. The causes of OA (which we will discuss below) are complex, multiple, and not always fully understood. Finally, doctors distinguish between primary OA (commonly called wear-and-tear arthritis) and secondary OA, which has an outside cause but often with signs and symptoms similar to the primary type. The subject of this chapter is primary OA, but much of the information contained here may also be useful to secondary-OA suffers.

SIGNS AND SYMPTOMS

Doctors identify disease by asking questions about a patient's history. They are looking for symptoms or subjective complaints of disease presence—what you feel in your knee. Common symptoms of OA include pain associated with weight bearing (like standing or walking), loss of motion, fatigue and decreased function, stiffness, looseness, giving way, throbbing, tenderness, and grinding or catching during knee movement.

Signs are the indicators of disease that your doctor can objectively verify. Some signs can be evaluated superficially, while others require the use of more sophisticated diagnostic tools that will be discussed in the next chapter. Among the arthritic signs that your doctor can observe by sight and touch are swelling, discoloration, the presence of scars and deformity, loss of motion, crunching with movement, loss of stability, and temperature changes around the knee. Tender reactive new bone accumulation (spurs or osteophytes) may form adjacent to the joint line as a result of abnormal stresses. These signs can occur as a result of the progressive deterioration of the articular cartilage and the pathologic changes that affect the surrounding structures. Based on experience, doctors can hypothesize about cartilage loss in the presence of the signs described above, but they will need to evaluate the inside of your knee to confirm this supposition.

THE STAGES OF ARTHRITIS AND PROGNOSIS

As a degenerative disease, arthritis develops along a continuum. It seems intuitive that the less advanced the stage of OA, the better the prognosis, or outlook, will be. Mild arthritis is the earliest phase of the disease and, if the proper steps are taken in time, the disease may not progress further. Mild OA is marked by occasional discomfort or minimal pain in the knee during or immediately after physically challenging activities, such as running, jumping, or climbing. It may be accompanied by mild inflammation or temporary impairment of the knee but on the whole will not have a major impact on how you live. Consider mild arthritis a warning sign that you need to make some adjustments to your lifestyle.

In moderate OA you may notice the same symptoms as in mild arthritis but of greater magnitude. Periods of joint pain and discomfort may be prolonged or be more intense and associated with stiffness and swelling that may occur twelve to twenty-four hours later. In addition, there will be a greater impact on your activities of daily living (ADLs). Prolonged engagement in some day-to-day activities, such as dressing, walking, or keeping house, may provoke symptoms and signs. The joint may not operate properly, prompting you to limp. You or your doctor may notice a decline in your physical capacity. In such a scenario the prognosis is guarded. If remedial action is taken, then the progression of the disease may be slowed. If changes in lifestyle are not made, then a progressive deterioration of the knee will occur.

Many of the signs and symptoms described above become chronic or more intense in severe, or late-stage, arthritis. Pain and often inflammation can be constant and debilitating. Even normal activities, such as standing or walking for even a few minutes, may be painful. Heat is sometimes felt. In some cases, the joint may become deformed and swollen. Hyaline cartilage has become so eroded that doctors call this state bone-on-bone arthritis. Immobility is the result in some cases. The prognosis is poor. Total joint replacement may be required.

CAUSES AND PATTERNS

Before we can fully understand any disease we have to investigate its causes. Knee OA, as we have seen, is a complex disease that afflicts an intricate joint, so it should come as no surprise that its causes are also complicated. In the most simplistic terms, knee OA is a wearing away of the hyaline cartilage that protects the bones that converge in the area we know as the knee. The result is usually some combination of pain and inflammation that ends in diminished functionality of the joint. In searching for causes, we identify factors or events that directly or indirectly wear down cartilage.

Probably the most important cause of knee OA is what we have already described as excessive and repetitive impact loading. Just like the best-engineered moving parts of a machine, the components of your knee joint, often starting with cartilage, will wear out progressively with time and excess use. If these same motions are performed in the presence of added weight or impact, the effects are multiplied, as we learned in our discussion of biomechanics in the last chapter. Unlike inanimate machines, however, humans are capable of healing. Also, the rate that we wear out is influenced not only by our lifestyle choices but also by our genetics. We all eventually fall apart and die, but why rush it? Do you remember that the impact of normal walking alone creates a force load equal to five times your body weight across your knees? In other words, anything that increases weight or impact can be a contributing factor to the development of knee OA. In North America, excessive weight is a widespread problem, so it should come as no surprise that obesity is one of the leading causes of the destruction of hyaline cartilage. But just because you're skinny doesn't mean you won't get arthritic knees. If your job involves performing the same joint-stressing motions over and over, or carrying weight, or both, you are also a candidate. Many sports increase the stress on your knees and have the same effect. In some cases, the impact on the articular cartilage may be traumatic in nature. Point loading of knee cartilage in either single or repeated traumatic episodes explains why arthritis can be seen in only one knee. In other cases, however, loading is symmetrical, and arthritis can be found in the same stage of development in both knees. Because the joints of the lower extremity are exposed to far greater biomechanical forces during weight bearing than the upper half of the body, we see more arthritis of the hips and knees than of the shoulders and elbows. The famous Framingham Study suggested that heavy physical activities encountered on the job can cause anywhere from 15 to 30 percent of knee OA in men.

Arthritis can also develop indirectly as the result of damage to a part of the joint other than the hyaline cartilage. You may remember the menisci from the last chapter. They function as shock absorbers, stabilizers, and lubricators of your hyaline cartilage. A meniscus can be torn traumatically, resulting in functional loss. After meniscal loss (whether as a result of injury or surgical removal), a progressive deterioration of the knee will occur. You can also rip your ligaments. Remember that their job is to guide the joints of the knee through their proper motions. If they are thrown out of kilter by injury, they may distort the normal motion of the knee, again causing dangerous erosion of the hyaline cartilage.

The knee joint works as a tightly coordinated and finely tuned machine, so a shortcoming or a flaw in any part of the machine will eventually lead to malfunction of the whole system. We saw in chapter one that the quadriceps muscles not only power the motion of the knee but also serve to dampen the shock and stress under which the joint is constantly placed. Strengthening the quadriceps and hamstrings can decrease the ground reaction force by approximately 20 percent. One of the consequences of our sedentary lifestyles is deconditioned or weak muscle. If we don't keep muscles strong, they are unable to lessen the effects of weight and impact on our bones and cartilage. The result is deterioration, or arthritis.

Decreased production of hyaluronic acid as a result of knee OA is another defect in the system that can have disastrous consequences. We can think of hyaluronic acid as a slippery ingredient of normal synovial fluid, which lubricates cartilage and other parts of the joint so as to ensure smooth movement. If this fluid is not produced in sufficient quantity or quality, the result will be deficient cartilage, which is prone to deterioration.

A final cause of arthritis has less to do with what we do than who we are. It is a reality of our biological existence that each one of us is a little different. Some are big and some are small. Some have bad eyesight or hearing. And some of us have been endowed with better cartilage than others. As with so many diseases, with arthritis too it appears that some people are genetically predisposed. On an almost equally fatalistic note, pathologic hormonal changes that take place in the body can sometimes be to blame. Diabetes and certain thyroid disorders may be linked to genetic transmission. But it's not all bad news. Such variables are just two among many risk factors leading to knee OA. By making changes in areas of your life that you do have control over, you can decrease your overall risk of developing arthritis. Nutritional supplements are one very simple way of fighting back that I will discuss at greater length later in the book.

FREQUENCY AND DEVELOPMENT OF KNEE OA

According to the US Centers for Disease Control (CDC), symptomatic knee arthritis occurs in at least 12 percent of people over the age of sixty, with a higher rate in females. Almost 50 percent of people will develop symptomatic knee arthritis by the age of eighty-five. Two out of three people who are obese will develop degeneration of the knee. Based on well-performed unbiased epidemiological (incidence, distribution, and possible control of disease) studies, heavy weight-bearing occupations, such as farming and mining, will lead to a much higher incidence of knee arthritis. Indeed, jobs that require excessive squatting, bending, kneeling, and stair climbing predispose to the onset of knee arthritis. Certainly those who have had significant injuries to their knees, such as a meniscal or ACL tear, are more likely to develop knee arthritis, even despite treatment that is now available.

THE IMPACT OF ARTHRITIS ON YOUR LIFESTYLE

Imagine living a painful, lonely life with no easy way to get around—that's the reality of living with untreated knee OA. Most of us want to live life to its fullest. Knee OA, when advanced, restricts us from physically achieving pain-free walking and full functional independence. Arthritis can significantly impact our everyday lives not only by altering the normal function of our knees but also by causing pain. Stiffness and loss of motion associated with swelling and deformity can produce pain. The pain further restricts motion. Eventually, even simple acts like putting on socks can be almost impossible. Although walking may be difficult, kneeling and stair climbing can be a major challenge. Even while lying in bed, pain may be your unwanted companion, resulting in lost sleep. Insomnia gives birth to progressive exhaustion and consequent loss of focus and memory, not to mention personality changes, such as nastiness. As knee OA worsens, the ensuing disability may require knee braces and a cane, making a handicap placard a necessity. In an attempt to control pain, some patients may turn to alcohol and prescription narcotics. Addiction and alcoholism further complicate and worsen the outlook for people with knee OA.

WHAT ARTHRITIS IS NOT: OSTEOPOROSIS

Many of my patients confuse osteoarthritis with osteoporosis. Other than the fact that they both affect bones, there is no similarity. However, osteoarthritis may occur in the presence of osteoporosis. Because osteoporosis is such a major problem, it's worth discussing briefly—what it is, its causes, and prevention. Arthritis, as we've seen, causes the progressive destruction of joints. Osteoporosis affects the structure of the bone itself. The word osteoporosis is also derived from Greek: *osteo*, you may remember, means "bone," while *porosis* means "the condition of being porous." When young and healthy, the femur, for example, is like a tube, with thick, dense, and solid walls possessing great strength, like an oak tree. With osteoporosis, the walls of the femur become thin, porous, and weak, like balsa wood. The osteoporotic bones break or fracture much easier than healthy bones. Progressive bone loss generally begins around the age of forty. The rate of bone loss significantly increases after fifty. In women, the progressive loss of bone after menopause is still more dramatic. The condition is diagnosed using bone densitometry, a painless x-ray study ordered by your physician.

The causes of osteoporosis are complex, but we do know that keeping your bones strong when young decreases the probability that you will develop osteoporosis. How do you keep and maintain bone strength? Exercise and proper diet are important in youth and as we age. Regular weight-bearing activities such as walking and weight lifting combined with a well-balanced diet containing adequate vitamin D and calcium are important to build and maintain bone strength. In northern latitudes, exposure to sunlight on a regular basis is important. In postmenopausal women, calcium and vitamin D supplements should be taken. Cigarette smoking and drinking carbonated beverages can lead to osteoporosis and should be stopped.

It has been observed that we enter life through the ring of the pelvis and exit through the neck of the femur. This remains true. We are usually born through the pelvic birth canal and may succumb to death following a fractured hip. The biggest cause of these fractures is trauma in the presence of osteoporosis, which has caused the bones to weaken. The bones most commonly broken are the hip, radius, and vertebra. In the United States alone there are approximately 300,000 hip fractures, 600,000 wrist fractures, and 750,000 vertebral compression fractures per year. The financial burden is huge, and the human toll incalculable. About one-third of women and one-fifth of men will develop osteoporosis as they age.

EVALUATING THE KNEE: PHYSICAL EXAMINATION AND IMAGING

When an orthopedic surgeon evaluates a patient's knee, he or she does so in a systematic fashion. First, we observe the way a person walks. Is there a limp? Is one leg shorter than the other? The knee is then inspected visually. We look at the knee to see if scars are present. There may be swelling and possibly even fluid accumulation. Discoloration such as redness or bruising is noted. The knee may be deformed or crooked. It's not uncommon to see a bow-legged or knock-kneed deformity in late-stage arthritis. The patient may hold the knee in a bent or contracted position. It may be "locked," suggesting a loose body or displaced cartilage caught in the joint. Chronic inactivity or guarding against painful motion may cause the thigh muscles to waste away or atrophy. Motion of the knee is carefully examined. The kneecap may deviate from its groove during bending, or even dislocate.

In addition, the doctor will palpate, or touch, the knee. The physician feels for increased warmth in the joint. As the knee is moved actively from extension into flexion, a *crepitus*, or crunching, may be felt along the joint surfaces, suggesting a wearing away of the articular cartilage. "Water on the knee" (synovial effusion) can also be felt.

Muscle tone and power are assessed to determine if the muscles are losing their strength. By holding and stressing the knee, the doctor can determine if the knee is unstable or loose. There are specialized stress tests to examine the anterior and posterior cruciate ligaments, as well as the collateral ligaments. The doctor may even listen to the knee. Sometimes, while a knee is being bent, a snap can be heard. During active flexion and extension, your doctor may listen for a crunching sound.

After carefully hearing the complaints of the patient and conducting a thorough physical examination, the doctor is prepared to order diagnostics (lab tests) and imaging studies (such as x-rays, CT scans, ultrasounds, and MRIs). Here, we will discuss three of these options: x-rays, CTs, and MRIs.

A type of ionizing radiation called an x-ray is often used to evaluate knee problems resulting from arthritis or injury. X-rays can result in harmful effects on the human body if used excessively. Fortunately, with newer types of x-ray tubes, the dose of radiation is minimized. X-rays are used to get an inside view of bones around the knee. The x-ray tube is directed at the knee, and the image is captured on special film. Nowadays, x-rays are captured in a digitized format called PACS (picture archival and communications systems) medical-imaging technology. Until about ten years ago, an orthopedic surgeon would "flip" an x-ray film up on a light box for review. The x-ray is now examined on a computer screen.

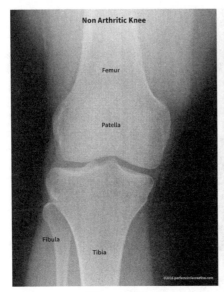 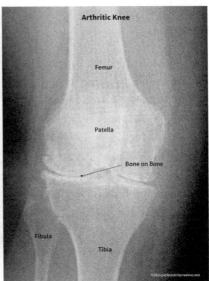

Diagram 9 **Diagram 10**

A variation of the x-ray is the CT scan (computerized tomography). CT scans consist of multiple x-ray cross sections of the body that are formatted using a computer to give two- and three-dimensional images. This allows doctors to more accurately evaluate the bone architecture. Difficult-to-evaluate fractures and deforming arthritis can now be assessed in great detail. The downside of CT scans is that more ionizing radiation is used than with standard x-rays. The femur, tibia, and patella all have characteristic images on x-rays (see diagram 9).

X-rays look primarily at the bone and not at soft tissue. Swelling of the soft tissues can be seen, although not with any detail; the doctor cannot determine, for instance, whether there is water or blood in the knee. Furthermore, the doctor cannot tell from an x-ray whether an infectious process is occurring or a noninfectious inflammatory condition. Characteristic x-ray changes seen in the knee as a result of arthritis include (1) narrowing of the joint space (wearing away of the hyaline cartilage and or meniscal cartilage [see diagram 10]); (2) whitening (hardening) of the bone adjacent to the articular cartilage loss; (3) reactive benign inflammatory bone cysts within the bone; and (4) bone spur (osteophyte) formation adjacent to the joint surface. These are often felt as tender ridges of bone on the medial or lateral aspect of the joint and are referred to as marginal osteophytes. When they are large, they can restrict motion of the knee and cause pain.

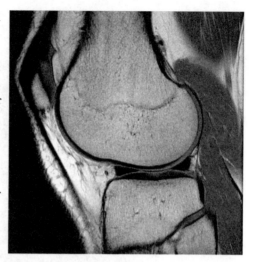

Diagram 11

A major advance in the diagnosis of knee problems occurred in the 1980s. With the introduction of the MRI (magnetic resonance imaging), doctors could more accurately diagnose disease and trauma within the knee. MRIs require a significant amount of time to complete (often up to 45 minutes per study). Because they use no ionizing radiation, they do not harm the patient (see diagram 11).

Some newer MRI machines are open and better tolerated by people with claustrophobia. The MRI images are captured digitally and can be conveniently transported over the Internet or on CDs for the doctor to read. Radiologists who are specially trained in the interpretation of MRIs read the images.

Many patients with moderately advanced or severe arthritis do not require an MRI, as x-rays adequately assess the degree of arthritic change. These expensive studies should only be ordered when they will alter treatment of a knee problem. For example, if the patient presents to a physician's office with only mild knee discomfort and no catching or locking, then a physical examination and x-rays may be enough to make an accurate diagnosis and set up a treatment program. However, if the patient presents to the office with an x-ray suggesting mild to moderate arthritis in the presence of catching or giving way, often an MRI will be used to determine if a displaceable cartilage tear is present. Displaceable cartilage tears can result in progressive joint damage if untreated. They can act like shards of metal in a ball-bearing joint, resulting in eventual destruction of the fine surface. Fortunately, with the invention of microsurgical techniques using arthroscopy, such tears can be treated on a daycare basis, using tiny incisions with little pain, and yield encouraging results.

PART TWO

TREATING KNEE ARTHRITIS— TAKING BACK YOUR MOBILITY

CHAPTER 3

BIOMECHANICAL TREATMENT

In the first two chapters we looked at the anatomy and function of the knee itself and at how arthritis develops and affects knee health. In the chapters that follow I would like to consider ways of treating knee arthritis before moving on to the final section of the book, where I will discuss how you can maintain knee health once it has been achieved through treatment. The challenge, in some ways, is to break a vicious circle; unchecked mild arthritis will eventually lead to moderate and severe arthritis. As protective cartilage is worn away, more bone is exposed. This leads to increased pain. A natural reaction to pain is decreased movement, but the consequence of less movement is muscle and ligament weakening and deconditioning. Which takes us back to square one, as we saw in chapter two. We will begin chapter three with a look at treatments that are informed by a basic understanding of biomechanics and are accessible to anyone. Then in chapters three and four, we will consider physical therapy and pharmaceuticals as further treatment approaches.

They call it the practice of medicine, and "practice makes perfect." My patients challenge me constantly with statements like, "I don't want to use drugs because they 'cover up' the pain." By this I think they mean that the drug doesn't cure the cause of the pain but rather masks the symptoms. In many instances, this is true. For example, non-steroidal anti-inflammatory drugs (NSAIDs) decrease the pain and inflammation of arthritis, thus allowing patients to overly stress already arthritic joints, thereby increasing damage to the articular surface. So if medication alone is used in the treatment of knee arthritis, acceleration of joint deterioration may result. Medication, which we will discuss later, must be used as part of a multipronged attack on the cause of arthritic symptoms. Drugs should be combined with weight loss, strengthening, and the other conservative measures that we are considering in this chapter.

WALKING ACCOMMODATIONS

It is logical to start with a short discussion of the most basic biomechanical "treatments." These are instinctive reactions to pain or malfunction that everyone has and can be called walking accommodations. Limping is an obvious example of a protective accommodation. I think of Festus in the TV series *Gunsmoke*. He had been shot in the leg at some point. Whenever his leg acted up, he would walk with a painful lurch. During a limp, the body leans to the affected side. By doing so, less force is placed over the arthritic joint. This protective mechanism shields the knee from the force of walking. A similar effect is seen when someone with an arthritic knee is standing. Weight is kept off the arthritic knee, which is held in a comfortable bent position, while most of the weight is put on the healthy leg.

Another accommodative change that can be used to decrease the symptoms of knee arthritis is gait retraining. Our gait is the manner in which we walk. By externally rotating the arthritic leg (that is, turning your toes to the outside), less stress is placed across the medial aspect of the knee. This results in less medial compartment arthritic pain. Also, by walking more slowly, less stress is placed across the knee joint. When we walk fast, generally our heel strikes the ground firmly, resulting in an increased ground reaction force jolting up the leg to the knee. That's why I tell my patients to walk carefully and deliberately—like a ninja.

FOOTWEAR

Bioengineers have also studied the effects of shoes on the ground reaction force. Did you know that high-heel shoes can increase the force across the knee by almost 20 percent? Scientists have discovered that the best shoes for someone with knee arthritis are thin-soled and flexible. Current evidence suggests that walking barefoot results in the lowest stress felt by the knee. This may be because without shoes we are more aware of the ground reaction force and tend to walk softly. I don't know about you, but you won't catch me walking city streets barefoot in the summer, let alone in January.

Over the years, doctors have tried heel wedges to decrease the amount of stress on arthritic knees. Although appealing, recent carefully performed studies suggest that wedges are of no apparent value in the treatment of knee arthritis. Beware of other gadgets that salesmen try to sell you on TV or online for treatment of your knee arthritis. No matter how convincing they sound, salesmen are not interested in you. In my view, heel wedges and other such contrivances are just another way of driving a wedge between you and your hard-earned money. Flexible and flat anatomic shoes are affordable and will make it easier for you to walk slowly and smoothly without driving your heels into the ground.

WALKING WITH A CANE

I said above that limping and gait correction were instinctive, or natural, walking accommodations. Often the most useful technologies are the simplest improvements on such natural reactions. The cane is a simple little tool that will take you a big step beyond limping and gait correction. When used correctly, a cane can significantly reduce the ground reaction force across your knee.

In order for a cane to be useful, it has to fit properly. Grasp the handle of the cane while standing normally, with your hands comfortably hanging at your sides so that your elbow is bent at about twenty degrees. The tip of the cane should be approximately four inches from the outside edge of your foot. Hold the cane in the hand opposite the side of the knee arthritis. "What?" you say. "That's not how Dr. House held it on TV!" Precisely. He was a brilliant and eccentric physician, addicted to prescription drugs, who used his complaints of arthritis as a tool to obtain narcotics. Unfortunately, he did not have a sound basis in biomechanics like you. If he did, he'd have held the cane in his opposite hand and decrease the pain of arthritis dramatically. What happens if you hold the cane in the hand that is on the same side as the knee arthritis? You increase the stress across the arthritic knee by approximately 20 percent. It would be better, under this circumstance, never to have used the cane unless, of course, you are looking for sympathy.

Let's take a minute to look at how a cane works, because it's not as obvious as it might at first appear. In reality, there are two underlying principles in the use of a cane. First, the walking-assist decreases the joint force crossing the opposite knee joint. Think of it like this: when you push down on the ground with a cane you weigh less. Prove this to yourself. Stand on a scale without using a cane and see how much you weigh. Then push down on the ground with the cane and see what the scale reads—it's less. It's similar to using a railing when climbing stairs. By holding the railing, you not only pull yourself up the stairs, but you also decrease your essential weight. A cane works in the same way. When held in the opposite hand, a cane decreases the amount of weight that crosses the knee joint.

Second, the use of a cane decreases what orthopedic surgeons call the adduction moment across the opposite knee. When walking, you are dynamic, or moving. Increased bending stresses are placed on your knees during walking. The most common form of arthritis affects the medial, or inside, compartment of the knee. As the articular cartilage wears away asymmetrically, a bow-legged (varus) deformity results (see diagram 5). In a knee with medial compartment arthritis a person becomes progressively bow-legged—like a cowboy who just climbed off his horse. In the knee too, a greater varus angulation causes increased joint force to go through the medial aspect of the knee when standing, resulting in more symptoms. As the knee "falls into varus," instability also occurs because of cartilage loss (a reverse shim effect) and loosening of the ligaments. When walking, the dynamic joint stresses escalate even more because of the increased bending force. Because of the bow-legged deformity and instability, patients with medial compartment arthritis may walk with a limp. When their heel hits the ground and the leg is loaded, the knee suddenly bends outward (varus thrust). Watching someone walk, an experienced eye can spot medial compartment arthritis a mile away. A cane helps by shifting the weight off the arthritic medial compartment to the normal lateral aspect of the knee, resulting in less force across the diseased area. The effect? Lessening of the lurch and decreased pain while walking. This means you can walk farther with fewer symptoms. You can also bend your knee more and strengthen muscles—both good things.

So if canes work so great, why aren't more people using them? Well, there's this thing called vanity. Many of my patients seem to think that a walking-assist makes them look "crippled." Not me! I look on it as a badge of courage. Those who use canes are not afraid to admit to themselves and others that they have arthritis, and they won't let it slow them down. And a cane can be a thing of beauty. Several of my patients have gifted me with intricately carved walking sticks, which work just as well as the aluminum cane from the pharmacy. I remember visiting my grandparents in Hawkestone, Ontario, as a little boy and seeing a canister by the front door. It was filled with around fifteen different canes used by my grandfather, who suffered from arthritis. Each was handmade, beautiful, and had a story to tell. Some were made from plain hickory with branch knobs still present, while others were hand-engraved. You see, in the old days, surgery was not an option. And a cane can make you look distinguished—think of Fred Astaire.

The therapeutic effects of cane use may not occur immediately. Some studies suggest that it takes well over a month for a cane to lessen arthritic symptoms. It is an easy, cost-effective way to treat arthritis. It can give you back your life. And if anyone gives you grief, they should beware. As all sheep and bad actors know, the cane can be used as a means of correction.

BRACING

Bracing is another simple measure that can decrease the force across the knee joint. Unloader braces are a popular way of treating mild to moderate medial compartment arthritis. They dynamically "straighten" the knee by putting stress at three points across the knee joint. It's like a hand pushing against the outer portion of the knee joint while two other hands push first against the inner aspect of the mid-thigh and second against the inner aspect of the mid-calf—resulting in a correction of the bowlegged deformity. As a consequence of the bracing, less pressure is placed across the medial aspect of the knee, which results in less pain from arthritis. Recent orthopedic studies have suggested that medial-lateral hinge-knee braces are as effective as unloader braces. These simpler braces are much less expensive than the unloaders and better tolerated. Although braces can be quite effective, the problem is that they often wind up in the closet because they are uncomfortable to wear. Wearing a hot, sweaty brace in summer is not reasonable. Under such conditions, braces are poorly tolerated and are a cruel and unusual form of punishment.

MUSCLE STRENGTHENING

I have already mentioned several times that muscles dampen the loads placed on the knee and protect and maintain the bearing surface. By strengthening the muscles in your legs—particularly the quadriceps—you can make a significant contribution to the health of your knee joints. This can be done simply by staying active in little everyday ways—taking the stairs instead of the elevator, walking short distances rather than driving your car, and devoting a few minutes every day to sports or exercise. In the next chapter we will look at physical therapy as a treatment approach, and there I will have more to say about muscle strengthening.

THE IMPORTANCE OF WEIGHT LOSS

Don't you just hate getting on the scale after Thanksgiving dinner? The reading reflects the gravitational pull on your body mass, but it always seems like someone turned the gravity up after the holiday, doesn't it? Most of us dislike discussing our weight because we'd prefer to be thinner. Aside from the negative self-image, weight loss is necessary to decrease stress on arthritic knees. And we're always confronted with that unpleasant dilemma that accompanies the decision to try to lose weight: eat less or exercise more. No one ever said losing weight was fun, but if you are overweight and want to be free of your arthritic symptoms, this is the single most effective step you can take.

As a man, I can safely say that most middle-aged guys give very little thought to diet. They eat when hungry and drink when thirsty. Freedom! A loss in weight corresponds to a loss in strength—and only the strong survive. In our younger years, when we were more active, physically and hormonally, weight took care of itself. Young athletes can pretty much eat whatever they want and not gain weight. We see these young bucks on the beach sporting biceps and six-pack abs. They move with the self-confidence of Adonis. As we advance in age, the pounds are not so easily shed, especially since our dietary habits are often still those established in our youth. But as we age, we don't burn calories like we did in our teens. As a consequence, we often find ourselves with a middle-age paunch when we reach the age of forty. This gut can be as hard to shake as a repo man.

But the problem isn't just age. Over the last six decades, there's been a tremendous change in the physical shape not only of Americans but also of many people throughout the industrialized world. Prior to 1950, the great majority of people were thin by our current standards. However, with advances in the availability of food and the dramatic changes in the composition and preparation of it, together with the decreased physicality of people, we have witnessed a gradual expansion of our waistlines. Most recent estimates suggest that in the United States, approximately 70 percent of men and 60 percent of women are overweight. Guys! One-third of us are obese! I recently watched the original film version of *The Grapes of Wrath*, starring Henry Fonda. You will recall it tells the story of a family during the Great Depression who were driven from their home in Oklahoma and eventually settled in California. I was surprised to see how thin most of the actors were. And it wasn't just because times were hard economically. Around the same time, I was looking over a bunch of old photos of my family taken in the 1950s and was struck by the fact that everyone in the pictures was slim. Not so in recent times. People that I would've once viewed as fat, I now see as being of acceptable size. My eye has accommodated to looking at plumpness as normal. In my opinion, the majority of obesity in the United States has a behavioral rather than organic cause. Before embarking on a weight loss program, it is prudent to undergo a physical exam to rule out other causes of weight gain, such as metabolic diseases.

How many patients have asked me if I could prescribe a weight loss pill? Many. Well, we had one that was very effective—Fen/Phen, an anti-obesity medication consisting of two anorectic drugs. And it worked well—if it didn't kill you. It also caused valvular heart disease and pulmonary hypertension, both life-threatening conditions. The FDA took the drug off the market in 1997. Two classes of drugs are commonly used to promote weight loss: appetite suppressants and fat-absorption inhibitors. We're talking about serious money here. Americans spend over $50 billion yearly on weight-loss products. The drugs, however, do not get to the root cause of weight gain. People with a weight problem need counseling, education, and a realistic program of diet and exercise. This involves work—a four-letter word. It is human nature to want a miracle weight-loss pill. Sadly, many over-the-counter weight-loss meds are nothing more than old-fashioned snake oil. Some can even cause damage. Like making money, it's best to lose weight the old-fashioned way—earn it.

Before we look at some healthier ways that you can start winning the "battle of the bulge," it's important to understand what it means to be overweight. Scientists who study weight have devised several methods for determining what a healthy weight is for people of all shapes and sizes. Let's take a quick look at a couple of those now.

WHAT IS MY HEALTHY WEIGHT?

The matter of healthy weight is actually quite complex. Adolphe Quetelet, a Belgian social scientist and mathematician who lived in the mid-1800s, wanted to design a mathematical model that would categorize a person's weight as compared to that which was normal and expected. He noticed that a person's weight generally increased as the square of the height, and based on his observation, he invented a predictive equation describing this relationship. In 1972 his equation was named the body mass index (BMI). He used the metric system—kilograms for weight and meters for height. This was his equation:

$$BMI = \frac{mass}{height^2}$$

Quetelet studied a large group of people, recording their heights and weights. From his observations he formulated a table determining a normal BMI. Today we have labeled a BMI of 18.5 to 25 as acceptable. A BMI of greater than 25 is considered overweight. A BMI greater than 30 is considered obese.

I don't like the word "obese" because it can have a negative connotation. Overweight people stigmatized as obese are often socially ostracized as having poor impulse control, lacking self-discipline, being sloppy, etc. All of us are familiar with the derogatory terms often aimed at overweight people. Weight-based stereotypes are often applied as well to those who are thin. Insulting terms such as "anorexic," "scrawny," "excessive dieters," "compulsive exercisers," and "bulimic" are directed at them. As a healer and teacher, my goal is to help people, not insult them. Well-meaning humor is often the best medicine. With this in mind, I've introduced the unscientific Morley height/weight chart.

THE MORLEY HEIGHT/WEIGHT CHART (USING BMI)	
BMI	**Category**
18.5–25	Ideal
25–30	Prosperous
30–35	Chubbette
36–40	Chubbola
41–45	Wicked Chubbola

Not everybody buys into the BMI concept. I mean, your height and weight change as you age. Some physicians suggest that as we age our weight should increase. I disagree. As we age, we lose muscle mass and bone minerals. It is reasonable to conclude that we should tip the scales less. If we weigh more in our old age, it's usually because we are fatter. Adiposity (fatness) is unhealthy at any age. Young and old alike should be slender. In addition, BMI charts do not take into consideration bone structure or frame. As a physician, I can pretty much assess someone's frame size by measuring the circumference of his or her wrists. Big wrists equal big bones. When I see a young man who is six foot two and 250 pounds with large wrists, I think, farm-boy big! Quetelet wanted to quantify "fatness" in moderately sedentary average people. The problem is that the BMI concept falls apart when considering muscular athletes. Muscle weighs substantially more than fat and takes up less room. Arnold Schwarzenegger, when he won the Mr. Universe title, would have been classified as "morbidly obese," according to BMI charts, which of course is ludicrous.

BMI does not take into consideration the distribution of fat. Increased abdominal or truncal fat, affectionately called the "middle-age spread," is commonly seen as we age. You may have heard it called a beer belly, pot belly, or an apple shape. This is what doctors call central obesity and is associated with diabetes and heart disease. A "pear-shaped" configuration, or fat deposition in the butt and thighs, may be more forgiving with respect to the cardiac and endocrine systems. However, it is the *amount* of weight, not its distribution, that stresses the knees, predisposing people to—and worsening—arthritis.

There are alternatives to the BMI approach. Body composition is calculated using body-fat measurements that commonly include skin-fold caliper techniques and hydrostatic weighing. In the skin-fold caliper method, a pinch of waist fat is measured and compared to a chart that takes into consideration sex and age. Although easy to perform, it can be inaccurate. In hydrostatic weighing, a person is dunked in a pool and asked to exhale. Using the old principle of Archimedes—eureka!—you have a very accurate read-out classified as the gold standard of body-composition measurement. There are other methods, uncommonly used, such as the DXA scan, which can be very precise. However, of all these methods, the BMI chart, although approximately 150 years old, still yields a fast, if not necessarily precise, estimate as to whether a person is overweight.

Finally, the National Institutes of Health (NIH) has come up with a formula for calculating the ideal weight for both men and women. I share it not to humiliate you but to encourage you to strive after a goal. As an old friend of mine once said, "This table bites." The truth hurts, they say. But it is also said that it will set you free (hopefully from many pounds).

THE SIMPLE NIH IDEAL WEIGHT FORMULA

Adult man: 106 pounds for the first five feet of height and six pounds for each additional inch.

Adult woman: 100 pounds for the first five feet of height and five pounds for each additional inch.

We've covered a lot of ground quickly, so let's try to put it all together. I've assembled a table that may help in applying our understanding of biomechanics to the treatment of knee arthritis.

BIOMECHANICAL TREATMENT OF ARTHRITIS

Weight loss

Muscle strengthening

Use of a cane

Walking accommodations

Proper footwear

Bracing

METABOLISM: THE BURN

Jack Sprat could eat no fat.
His wife could eat no lean.
And so between them both, you see,
They licked the platter clean.

Metabolism, when used in a medical context, refers to a series of complex chemical reactions occurring in the body that make life possible. When a normal person uses the word, he or she usually is referring to a person's ability to burn calories. For our practical purposes, metabolism can be called "the burn." To give an example, when we say, "Joe has a great metabolism," we mean that he can eat like a horse and lose weight. Or if we say, "Susan has a slow metabolism," we mean that she puts on weight when eating like a bird.

The body is made up of trillions of cells, or units. Each cell has within it many little engines called mitochondria. The mitochondrial generators, as they burn fuel, supply the energy that powers each cell. All of these trillions of independent engines, chugging away together, allow the body to function as a whole complex machine. The sum total of the energy used to drive these trillions of little motors is metabolism. A calorie is a measurement of thermal energy or heat. It is the energy required to raise one gram of water one degree centigrade. We all know from experience that if you work hard physically—say, running or bicycling—you become hot and sweaty. What you're feeling is the "the burn." The fleet of mitochondrial engines produce heat as they rev. You sweat to cool down the big motor that is your body. Like a Prius, some people are genetically endowed to get more miles per gallon. Others have extreme metabolic needs and go through fuel like a 1967 Corvette Stingray with a 427 big-block tri-power V-8; they can scarf down a whole pizza, wash it down with a mug of root beer, and still have room for dessert without gaining weight.

Your body works like a complex city. Areas of the city are being torn down (catabolic), while other blocks are being built (anabolic). Cells do the work. The fuel that drives the mitochondrial engines powering each cell is glucose, which we derive from food. Nutrition is usually delivered to your body by eating, and the food you eat needs to be broken down by the body before it can be used as fuel.

In another analogy, your body is like a woodstove. Wood is fuel for the stove. If you burn green wood and decrease or choke the air flow, you produce smoke and little heat. Creosote builds up and clogs the chimney. But if you put dry wood in the very same stove and open the damper (provide oxygen), a roaring fire with little smoke is produced, and it burns away the creosote. The stove's burn is like your metabolism. In order to convert your body into an efficient burning machine, you need to do two things—feed it good seasoned wood (healthy food) and open the damper (exercise). As we have seen, your body contains stores of fuel in the form of fat. Ideally, we want to convert your body into an efficient fat-burning machine so you can lose pounds to decrease the stress on your knees.

If you are interested in learning more about how you can make metabolism work to your advantage, I highly recommend reading *The Metabolism Advantage* by John Berardi, PhD. This book has strongly influenced my thinking on metabolism. Dr. Berardi explains that there are four components of metabolism: (1) resting metabolic rate (RMR); (2) physical-activity level (PAT); (3) energy cost of eating; and (4) genes. Even when you do nothing, you're burning calories. Your heart is beating, your lungs are breathing, your brain is active, and all the many essential functions required to maintain life are working. Believe it or not, just staying alive uses up the greatest portion of calories you use. Increasing physical activity burns more calories. Even eating uses up calories. As we shall see later in the book, food is made of macronutrients. The body processes different macronutrients in different ways, and some require the burning of more calories than others. Whatever the process, energy is expended. Finally, your genetic makeup is also a decisive factor; some people simply have more efficient metabolism than others.

The question of weight loss is complex. Some suggest that losing weight is simply a matter of taking in fewer calories. But it's not that simple. Ideally, the weight we want to lose is fat. If we starve ourselves, our body transforms itself into a high-efficiency machine by hunkering down on energy expenditure. It goes into "starvation mode." Even when starving, your body needs to keep the lights on. The fuel burned to maintain basic life is in the form of glucose. Glucose is produced preferentially from the breakdown of muscle rather than fat. In other words, when you starve, your muscles waste away. By drinking coffee all day, and then going into a feeding frenzy at night, you have fooled your body into starvation mode. As a result, you lose muscle mass during the day and store away fat after supper. With time you become a starving person trapped in a fat person's body. The correct behavior is to make breakfast your big meal. After all, you are breaking a night-long fast. Eating small portions of nutritious food every two to three hours maintains steady glucose levels, thereby maintaining muscle and inhibiting fat deposition. Dinner should be a small meal in early evening.

The matter of weight loss, which as a rule is a positive goal, is complicated by the consideration of the type of tissue being lost. Muscle, although more compact, weighs more than fat. So paradoxically, eating correctly and exercising may result in weight gain. Even though you will become trimmer practicing these healthy habits, the scale reads gravitational force, and volumetrically muscle weighs more than fat. In this case, it is okay to ignore the scale and focus on your waistline (and the admiring glances of your friends).

How we eat is a strong predictor of weight gain, but it too is a complex matter. We eat less when surrounded by friends. Drinking alcohol before a meal increases the amount we eat. Eating a small amount of protein or fat before the main meal—an hors d'oeuvre—decreases the overall calorie intake. The type of fuel or food we eat influences metabolism. Eating proportionally more protein than carbs and fat will result in weight loss. Protein burns hotter than carbohydrate or fat.

Here again we see that the matter is complex. You need fat to live! There's good fat and bad. Fat makes you feel full. Too much fat chokes the furnace. Eat good fats—olive oil, fish, free-range chicken, and grass-fed and grass-finished meat—in moderation. Eating more fiber in the form of healthy leafy veggies leads to weight loss. And all of the above is modified by activity level. Before vigorous exercise our body needs protein and carbs. Immediately after a workout, a hit of carb is necessary for muscle growth. Mother never said it would be easy.

But we're interested in turning up the burn. We can't alter our genes; those are the cards we've been dealt. We can, however, boost our resting metabolic rate (RMR) by increasing our lean muscle mass and improving flexibility. How do we do that? By applying Wolf's Law, which states that form follows function. When we do resistance and flexibility exercise and eat more protein, our muscles grow bigger. Muscle motors burn through fuel (i.e., food). And how about this: muscle burns calories not only when you exercise but also from twenty-four to forty-eight hours after a good workout—the "afterburn." You don't get this effect with a cardio workout; "you burn as you turn, and there's no afterburn." That's why resistance exercise is crucial in the maintenance of good health, muscle gain, and weight loss. Remember, weight loss and strong legs mean less arthritic knee pain. Don't succumb to Old Man Time. Work with weights (or do other muscle-building exercises), eat well, and increase overall muscle mass. This will lead to an increase in your resting metabolic rate. The added benefit is that you will feel and look younger and can eat more good food. And your knees will hurt less! I'll have more to say about both exercise and healthy eating later in the book. In the meantime, do your best to follow this simple weight loss formula. You can remember it with the acronym SVELTE.

Smaller meals

Veggies

Eat breakfast

Lots of protein

Take time for meals

Exercise

SPECIAL DIETS FOR WEIGHT LOSS

Americans want answers and results, and they want them now. The word *diet* comes from ancient Greek and means "way of living." In modern times it has come to denote not just a way of living but a way of eating to lose weight. And systems there are! Some work well—for a period of time. Some are bizarre. Others are sensible and easy to follow. Some are fraudulent and unhealthy. Many are expensive. Let's look at a few popular diets that may be able to help you get on the road to weight loss and a healthy, arthritis-free life.

I see most of the diets discussed here are as a first step along the road to healthy living; once you get your weight down to a reasonable level, it will be your job to make changes to your lifestyle that will enable you to keep it there. (These changes will be discussed in part three of this book.) What follows is meant to be a quick overview and is far from comprehensive. If a certain diet appeals to you, there are exhaustive materials available at the click of a mouse or at your local library.

THE ATKINS DIET

The Atkins diet was the first popular "low-carb" diet. Dr. Atkins, a cardiologist, launched the low-carb revolution in 1972. There are many theories as to why the Atkins diet works. Some say that the monotony of a protein/fat diet decreases the amount of overall caloric intake. Others have stated that the diet produces a "metabolic advantage." A diet that is low in carbohydrates has a low glycemic index. In other words, it does not drastically affect your blood sugar. We will discuss this at greater length in the section on nutrition, but suffice it to say that such foods tend not to leave you feeling hungry for more. Thus, in theory, someone on the Atkins diet will eat fewer calories because he or she is less hungry.

We also know that the energy cost of eating protein is higher than that of eating carbohydrates. In other words, you burn more calories eating protein than carbs. If you like meat, eggs, fish, and butter, you've found your diet; Atkins is a carnivore's delight. It has been my observation that the Atkins diet works better in men than women. I have witnessed firsthand the positive effects of this diet—weight loss, increase in HDL (high-density lipoprotein), and decrease in blood pressure. From a practical standpoint, sticking with the Atkins diet long-term can be difficult. Also, for vegetarians, the Atkins diet can be challenging, as plant-based protein is limited when compared to meat-based sources. For those interested in trying the Atkins diet, start with *Dr. Atkins New Diet Revolution* (2002).

THE SOUTH BEACH DIET

Dr. Arthur Agatston, another cardiologist, developed the South Beach diet. In essence, his diet is also a high-protein diet but encourages carbohydrates with a low glycemic index. The South Beach diet also allows healthy fat (unsaturated fat and omega-3 fatty acids) while prohibiting trans-fats and discouraging saturated fat. This seems to me like a sensible diet that can be continued long term without the dieter submitting to the boredom of an all-protein/fat diet. I've often thought of the South Beach diet as a kinder, gentler form of the Atkins diet. If you're interested in learning more, you can obtain *The South Beach Diet*, published in 2005 by Rodale Books.

THE PRITIKIN DIET

The Pritikin Program for Diet and Exercise was published in 1979 and outlined Nathan Pritikin's approach. He developed this diet based on research he did while investigating treatment for his own heart disease. He described his diet as "mankind's original meal plan." His method consisted of eating predominantly unrefined complex carbohydrates. It is a low-fat, high-carbohydrate type plan that severely restricts the consumption of animal protein. The Pritikin diet includes unprocessed vegetables, beans, whole grains, fruit, and occasional lean meats and seafood. Culinary herbs rich in phytonutrients are included. This healthy diet restricts fats and oils, alcohol, sweeteners, salts, and processed food. Beverages allowed include herbal tea and water. You're allowed three cups of tea or one eight-ounce cup of coffee daily. This seems somewhat arbitrary and unfair to me. I need three cups of coffee in the morning just to get going. I tried the Pritikin diet years ago for about a month. I found it to be severe and restrictive. It resulted in weight loss but unfortunately was accompanied by hunger pangs and generalized muscle weakness. There's no way I could complete a heavy workout munching on grass. Got protein? I personally don't have the motivation to continue on this draconian diet for any significant amount of time without falling off the wagon and walking into the nearest butcher shop.

THE ZONE DIET

With *Enter the Zone*, biochemist turned diet guru, Barry Sears, PhD, kicked off a mega-money-making multimedia enterprise based on quasi-scientific grounds. The premise of the diet is that ingesting macronutrients in the following proportions is optimal: 40 percent carbs; 30 percent protein; and 30 percent fat. The Zone advocates veggies over starch and smaller, more frequent portions, while avoiding sugar and saturated fats. Dr. Sears claims that the diet, when followed, results in hormonal balance and decreased inflammation. Food portions are broken down into "Zone Blocks." The diet is complex to follow. It violates the KISS (Keep it simple, stupid!) principle and is therefore suspect and, in most cases, destined to fail. There are many critics of the "science" behind the diet. Testimonial evidence (enthusiastic people who've lost weight), the weakest form of evidence, is used to validate its effectiveness. However, I must confess that I really like the before-and-after photos seen in the infomercials. These slick advertisements bark, with evangelistic fervor, that if I buy into a diet, workout, or dance routine, like the people on the screen, I could lose thirty pounds, tighten up, and grow killer abs.

That being said, the diet itself seems healthy enough, considering it demands that people consciously evaluate what they're putting in their bodies and eat smaller, more frequent portions consisting of nutritious food. It should come as no surprise that the Zone diet results in weight loss. If combined with an exercise program, positive results will be seen. But you don't need to "enter the Zone" to eat well and exercise.

JENNY CRAIG/WEIGHT WATCHERS/NUTRISYSTEM

If all you want to do is lose weight, then a "no-brainer" approach may work for you. These systems come replete with literature, Internet support, and, in some cases, "encounter groups." Encounter groups can be very effective— after all, misery loves company. The camaraderie of starving people is legendary. However, these systems do not teach you the principles behind purchasing, preparing, and eating good whole food. I've had experience with processed, prepackaged food—and I do not wish to repeat it. At Camp Lejeune, during basic training in the United States Marine Corps, I lived on K-rations for a period of time. If you're going on a forced march, this food is suitable, but with the exception of the bread pudding, most of the food was barely palatable. Without being unduly harsh, I categorize prepackaged, microwaveable food in the same category as K-rations. The food offered in these systems is expensive, highly processed, unsavory, and in some cases unhealthy. The portions are smaller and lead to weight loss by limiting caloric intake. But the expense of these "foods" alone prohibits their long-term use. Their unappealing presentation and unpalatable taste guarantees their failure as a sustainable dietary plan.

VEGETARIANISM/VEGANISM

The Vegetarian Society was founded in Manchester, England, in 1847. The word vegetarian is derived from the Latin verb *vegere*, "to be alive, lively." A vegan, or strict vegetarian, eats only plant-based foods. There are variations on the theme. A lacto-ovo vegetarian will also allow milk and egg products.

Vegetarians eat significantly lower amounts of saturated fat and less protein. Not surprisingly, a vegetarian diet significantly lowers the incidence of coronary artery disease. The vegan diet contains increased fiber and more of certain micronutrients/phytochemicals when compared to an omnivorous diet. Vegetarians, in general, have a lower BMI. Studies show that they have less high blood pressure, cardiac disease, type 2 diabetes, kidney disease, and dementia. Vegans, however, can be at risk for certain deficiencies, such as vitamin B12, iodine, and iron. These inadequacies can be corrected by taking supplements, however.

The decision to follow a vegetarian or vegan diet, it seems to me, can be supported by scientific evidence. Many also support the various forms of vegetarianism on moral grounds. After all, who would disagree that slaughterhouses are most unpleasant places? Plant-based foods can be quite delicious as well. But for me, a meat-free existence is too big a sacrifice to make. It just tastes too darn good.

THE CABBAGE SOUP DIET

There are many versions of this diet, including the original, hardcore, full-on CSD. In the classic plan, cabbage soup with low-calorie veggies (including onions, celery, and tomatoes), flavored with chicken or beef stock and spices, is eaten for one week—as much as you want! Believe me, by the second day you won't want much. If you've made a sacred pledge to the sun and stars, you'll stick with the diet and lose between one and two pounds per day. No mystery there: you've been eating less than 600 calories a day. You'll be weak from muscle loss (and occasionally from electrolyte imbalance if you have the common side effect of stomach cramps and diarrhea) and ravenously hungry. This fad diet put the "yo!" into the expression "yo-yo diet." If you're trying to fit into a tuxedo or prom dress, this may be the diet for you. Otherwise, avoid it like the plague. It's unhealthy and not sustainable.

CRON (CALORIC RESTRICTION WITH OPTIMAL NUTRITION) DIET

This diet is the brainchild of Dr. Roy Walford, a brilliant and eccentric pathologist whose claim to fame is research into the life extension of mice using caloric restriction and optimal nutrition (CRON). From his animal studies, he extrapolated a diet for humans. His research led him to advocate eating less food but of higher quality. From a purely analytical standpoint, this diet makes good sense. It is solid and based on concrete animal studies. It results in improvement of "biomarkers," including blood pressure, cholesterol and triglyceride levels, and glucose tolerance tests. Among its outcomes is predictable weight loss, and it has been shown to dramatically increase life expectancy in lab mice. The CRON diet has, in certain studies, demonstrated increased lifespan in primates as well. Dr. Walford successfully implemented the diet in humans during his biosphere experiments in the Arizona desert. The health of the biosphere subjects was improved, based on physical examination and lab studies. The good doctor wrote *Beyond the 120 Year Diet: How to Double Your Vital Years*, which I regard as a classic and well worth reading. In a sad, ironic twist, Walford himself died at the relatively young age of seventy-nine of amyotrophic lateral sclerosis (Lou Gehrig's disease). His legacy lives on through his daughter, Lisa, who continues to promote the diet through books of her own, as well as her leadership in the CR Society.

Walford argued that industrialized Western humans have developed societal diseases as a result of eating bad food and too much of it. What effects the diet will have on humans remains unclear. Time will tell. But it makes sense to me: eat less, eat highly nutritional food, and the outcome will be weight loss and improved health. It is not an easy diet to follow amid all the tasty temptations that surround us. I have no doubt that if followed by a modern-day Nazarite, this diet could well result in improved health and significant life extension. Living to be as old as Methuselah (969 years), however, is still out of reach. Although not a CRONie, I have applied the principles of Dr. Walford's approach to my personal diet. It appeals to my scientific and common sense and results in healthy weight loss, which means losing fat but not muscle mass. This is exactly what we want in the treatment of knee arthritis.

THE 2-DAY DIET

This diet is the most recent diet sweeping the world. Believe it or not, it's not just a fad but also the real deal. It's an approach to dieting based on the research of Dr. Michelle Harvie and Prof. Tony Howell in Manchester, England. It's simple. Two days a week you cut your dietary intake (i.e., caloric restriction). The other five days you eat the Mediterranean way—good lean meat, fish, olives, veggies, salad, whole-grain bread, fruit, and even a little wine.

The diet emerged from research done at the Genesis Cancer Prevention Center. Studies there examined how excessive weight influenced the likelihood of developing breast cancer. This led to a search for an effective weight-loss diet that was sustainable. Out of this research emerged the 2-Day Diet. I would encourage you to read the book, *The 2-Day Diet*. The approach is healthy and easy to implement. And because it's balanced, no supplements are needed.

Why only a two-day diet? Dr. Harvie found that most people are unable to stick with a 24/7 "theme diet" for very long. Ditching a diet results in a relapse to bad eating habits and leads to the phenomenon of yo-yo dieting— you know, weight gain and then weight loss, just like the Hollywood stars and politicians who fall off the diet wagon and then run off to a southern Utah spa to whip themselves back into good health. But two days is something most people have the willpower to manage. The other five days, there's no pressure. At the same time, the diet results in healthy weight loss (remember: hang on to muscle and lose fat). Weight loss is good for your vanity (you look better in front of the mirror) and health (less risk of heart disease, diabetes, cancer, Alzheimer's, and arthritis). On a practical level, Dr. Harvie asks dieters to set short- and long-term goals.

Let's think about this diet. It's simple to follow. It's affordable. It's healthy. It's tasty. It's not a fad diet. It gets lasting results. Of all the diets I've examined, it makes the most sense to me.

DIETS AND WEIGHT LOSS: CONCLUDING REMARKS

Your weight is important. From an orthopedic standpoint, increased weight puts added stress on weight-bearing joints—particularly the knees. Being overweight can lead to arthritis. Once arthritis is present, being overweight accelerates joint degeneration. But what's more, excess weight also negatively affects your general health.

The problem is that in order to lose weight, you need to diet. And as we all know, dieting seems so wrong. It involves self-control, restraint, and pain. Sins of commission are more fun than virtues of omission. In the land of the free and the home of the brave, we are geared to "Go! Go! Go!" Dieting is downright un-American. That's because dieting is the opposite of eating without restraint. Genetically, we are wired to eat to fullness in order to store up fat supplies to be used in times of need. In past millennia, we were not always guaranteed a steady source of food. Hunters and gatherers had to work hard for it. In the biblical book of Genesis, we learn that during the reign of the pharaohs in Egypt, there were seven years of plenty and seven years of starvation. Wise Joseph rose to fame because he built storehouses to hold the grain that would feed the people during the times of famine. The idea was extraordinary because it had been a historical rule of thumb that in times of plenty, you stuffed yourself in order to get through the times of dearth. Today, however, we have only days of plenty.

To help and encourage you, I have come up with a set of General Laws of Eating that illustrate what would-be dieters are up against.

1. Eating is fun—alone or with friends.

2. Eating is easy.

3. Anyone can eat—it's the only thing you can do as well when you're eighty as you could when you were eighteen.

4. Food tastes good; fattening food tastes great!

The list could go on. The point is that behind the urge to eat there are complex biological and social forces that we must learn to control. Losing weight by dieting is not easy, but it is possible.

So as not to end on such a dire note, let me share a few tricks you can use to help lose weight that don't require much effort. I like to think of them as caloric expenditure freebies, and I have made a convenient list of them for you at the end of this chapter. You can increase your rate of metabolism. We can trick our systems into "turning up the burn." By drinking six glasses of ice water daily you will increase energy expenditure, thus burning calories. Certain foods have the same effect. These include hot peppers or foods containing them, green tea (also a potent antioxidant), fish oil, and many protein-rich snacks (e.g., protein bars). Using these tricks you can lose weight without breaking a sweat. But where's the fun there? When you work out you build muscle, and every pound of new muscle burns approximately fifty calories per day to meet its energy needs. Just remember: build a fire and lose the tire.

INCREASING METABOLIC ACTIVITY
(TURNING UP THE BURN)

- Ice water   6 glasses daily
- Fish oil capsules   2 with each meal
- Capsaicin   with each meal
- Green tea   with each meal
- Protein snack or bar   at snack time

CHAPTER 4

PHYSICAL THERAPY FOR ARTHRITIS PATIENTS

In the last chapter we examined a whole host of ways that you can mitigate the effects of arthritis without necessarily seeing a doctor. The suggestions there can be summarized as a list of ways to relieve stress on your knee joints, thereby diminishing arthritis symptoms. This chapter is about more specific ways of healing damage inflicted by arthritis, training your body to work in such a way as to avoid future damage, and maintaining physical health—all under the guidance of an expert who has been trained in physical therapy.

LAND PROGRAM

As humans, we live most of our lives on the land. We stand, walk, climb stairs, and get around. We call these the activities of daily living. Our strong legs and flexible knees, in conjunction with good balance, allow us to perform complex physical activities—running up and down stairs, getting in and out of cars, and carrying groceries into the house. Our legs also allow us to perform complex and physically demanding athletics. On land, our legs must fight the force of gravity, the effect of which is markedly diminished in the water. Many people suffering from knee arthritis are unable to perform these basic tasks. A physical therapy (PT) land program, as opposed to a water program, consists of exercises that may simulate these everyday activities to various degrees. In cases where land-based exercise is painful, or in the absence of sufficient strength, water programs are used. These will be discussed in the second part of this chapter.

A land program essentially involves range-of-motion exercises (ROM) and progressive resistance exercises (PRE). If you are unable to tolerate a home exercise program, your doctor may prescribe PT. You may gain many benefits from seeing a therapist. The condition of your knee arthritis will be professionally assessed, and a program specific to your needs will be designed.

The amount of bend you have in your knee is referred to as the range of motion. An athletic young person may have knee range motion of zero to 150 degrees. As we age, we lose flexibility in our knees. Most middle-aged and older people have a range of motion of zero to 130 degrees, but we can get by with significantly less flexibility.

Let's look at some common day-to-day physical activities. In the United States, every step in a staircase usually has a seven-inch rise for an eleven-inch run. Flexing the knee to 90 degrees allows people to climb stairs. Getting in and out of a car, depending on the height of the seat and car, requires knee flexion of approximately 105 degrees. Normal walking requires knee flexion of about 60 degrees. Although some people might quibble, I would place functional flexibility at around zero to 120 degrees. More flex is better—no question. Loss of motion usually accompanies knee arthritis. Most people think of loss of motion as loss of flexion, but from a functional standpoint, full extension is more important than full flexion; inability to straighten your knee completely makes weight bearing more difficult, and your knee may have a tendency to give out, leading to falling and injury. So when you consider range of motion, think both extension and flexion.

Most likely, your physical therapist will start with non-weight-bearing exercises. Depending on the circumstances, the therapist may start with gentle passive range of motion (PROM). These are exercises designed not to cause pain. The maxim "No pain, no gain" goes out the window in the PROM phase. The therapist will move your knee through motion without your helping. That is what makes it passive. Later, a progressive program will be started that incorporates active assisted range of motion (AAROM). At this point, you will help the therapist to move your joint. Finally, you graduate to the last stage— active range of motion (AROM), where you do the work, and the therapist does the watching. At first, you will do range-of-motion exercises against only gravity. As you become stronger, different forms of resistance will be added during the knee motion. This progression illustrates the principles underlying

PT. The therapist begins with a very active role—teaching, training, and providing physical assistance—and then slowly retreats into the background as you regain the ability to control your body autonomously.

Your therapist may have you perform many types of activities. You may be asked to do quadriceps and hamstring stretches. You will be instructed in straight-leg raising. You'll be asked to do heel slides as well as heel cord stretches. Because proper motion of your hip is required in the normal function of your knee, your therapist also may include hip-stretching exercises. In all of these exercises, the aim is to restore range of motion.

After functional range of motion has been achieved, your therapist may start you on progressive resistance exercises (PREs). Many patients are started on a weight-bearing program. Your therapist will teach you how to do these exercises at home. My favorites include wall slides and toe raises. As your strength improves, you may wish to graduate to single-leg wall slides and toe raises. But be careful. If you experience knee pain, you are loading your joint excessively and should back off.

Your therapist may then advance you to the use of Thera-bands. These color-coded elastic bands come in various degrees of resistance. They are a light, portable way of taking your gym with you, allowing you to perform your exercise program virtually anywhere. Free weights are another possibility that promote not only strength but also balance and agility. There are also more complex technologies (like Nautilus and Cybex), but the problem with fancy machinery is that it is often nonfunctional, expensive, and nontransportable. Two more advanced exercise machines that I stand by are the Versa-climber and the Concept 2 Indoor Rower. Such machines may be incorporated into an advanced land-based physical therapy, but they also may be an appropriate part of a maintenance-oriented exercise program. For this reason, I have chosen to discuss them at greater length later in the book.

MODALITIES

Your physical therapist will often use what are known as modalities in the treatment of arthritis. This is a fancy word that denotes pathways or tools used in the treatment of knee arthritis. Modalities include thermal energy, electrotherapy, ultrasound, laser, and mechanical energy.

Much of the value of using these modalities stems from their ability to control pain and inflammation, which go hand in hand. If the pain/inflammation cycle can be broken, even momentarily, then an exercise program can be started. Pain is complex and multifactorial. In arthritis, we know that inflammation is part of the puzzle. So if inflammation can be minimized, often a decrease in pain will follow. Modalities may also result in the production of endorphins. Endorphins are narcotic-like neurotransmitters produced by your body—without a doctor's prescription or co-pay! These chemicals are produced in your pituitary gland, brain, and nervous system. Just like real narcotics, they interfere with pain signals and cause a euphoric "buzz." Maybe you've seen their effect on the serene-looking face of a long-distance runner who is enjoying a "runner's high." A range of activities that includes stress, sex, physical activity, and the consumption of spicy foods produce endorphins. So if you really want to get your endorphins up, on date night take your sweetheart on a fast walk, talk politics, and have a meal of hot tamales with Tabasco sauce, followed by a moon-light stroll. Olé! Endorphin-fest.

Let's take a quick look at how the most common modalities work.

THERMAL ENERGY AS THERAPY

Thermal energy, or heat energy, passes into our bodies in four ways. The first is direct transfer, or conduction; for example, putting an ice or hot pack directly on the skin. The second possibility is circulation, or convection. This might consist of a convection oven blowing heat directly on an area, but it could also be a whirlpool, which circulates heat around an arthritic knee. Radiation is a third way that thermal energy can be transferred. A heat lamp, for instance, applies radiation energy to an area. Finally, there is conversion of one energy form to another. Heat can be produced in tissue using various forms of energy, including electrical energy, sound energy, light energy, or mechanical energy (all of which we will look at in a few paragraphs).

As the knee joint is close to the skin surface, external temperature modalities applied can penetrate quickly to the inner structures. Ice is readily accessible and cheap. You don't need a doctor's prescription to obtain it, and you can apply it to your knee in a variety of ways. Many people put water in a Dixie cup, pop the cup in the freezer, and peel the top inch of the cup away once it's frozen. By gripping the cup, the ice can be applied in a circular manner to the front of the knee for an ice massage. Or you can use the Birds Eye treatment: apply a package of frozen peas to the front of the knee, contouring it around the kneecap to give uniform coolness to the joint. Some people use lima beans, since the bigger beans hold cold for a long period of time. Still others apply ice the way many athletic trainers do—by filling a Ziploc bag with ice chips and water (water helps diffuse the cold, transferring temperature twenty-five times faster than air). The ice bag is then spread around the front of the knee. Or, if you want to get fancy, you can pick up reusable ice packs from the pharmacy. Remember to always put a cloth buffer between the ice and your skin. Frostbite can cause severe soft tissue damage.

How does cold on your knee work? Cold decreases blood flow to your muscles and nerves. We New Englanders know what happens to your feet if you stand outside for any length of time during January. As they become progressively colder, you feel pain, followed by a dull ache as the blood slows, depriving your feet of oxygen. If you don't start to move, you next feel a pins-and-needles sensation as a result of progressive loss of nerve function. A burning tickling follows, and the final phase is numbness. At this point it's probably a good idea to get out of the cold and warm your feet before you develop frostbite—a freezing of your soft tissues associated with cellular death. The cold also affects muscles. They progressively lose their power to contract. If you've ever been hypothermic, you'll understand. Your muscles become progressively weaker and stiffer.

But what does any of this have to do with treating arthritis? The physical properties of cold can effectively treat arthritic symptoms. As sensory nerves become sluggish when cold, they conduct fewer pain signals to the brain, resulting in diminished pain. So cold is a valuable tool that can decrease arthritic pain. In addition, as a result of both the application of cold and elevation of the leg when you apply ice as treatment, arthritic swelling is often diminished. In acute situations, like trauma or an arthritic flare, we use RICE therapy: rest, ice, compression, and elevation. Also, if there is an element of muscle spasm, then cold can be used to "break" the spasm. Ice works just fine in chronic situations, such as osteoarthritis, as well. The cold not only decreases blood flow but slows cellular metabolism too, effectively minimizing the inflammatory component of arthritis.

Generally, it's safe to use ice for around twenty minutes but not more than thirty because of the risk of injury from frostbite. I once evaluated a young quarterback who had a knee injury treated on the sidelines with ice application for ninety minutes. He was unable to elevate his foot upwards ("foot drop") because of thermal injury to the common peroneal nerve. Fortunately, the nerve thawed, and he regained normal leg strength over the next sixty minutes, much to the relief of all involved.

Then there is heat. Heat increases the blood flow when applied to the skin by causing vasodilation of the arteries. The rush of blood brings "healing factors" to the knee. Heat increases flexibility of soft tissues. Heat also can be used for pain control and moderation of muscle spasm.

If ice is nice and heat is neat, using them both in sequence can be a marriage made in heaven. The Swedes have paired the two with the contrast bath. Sequential ten-minute periods of ice-heat-ice are applied to the knee and can result in prolonged analgesia and acceleration of healing. Some suggest that the alternate-temperature-induced vasoconstriction and vasodilatation, when performed sequentially, creates a pumping action that may help decrease swelling within the tissues.

ELECTROTHERAPY

Electricity can also be used to treat arthritis. A TENS (transcutaneous electrical nerve stimulation) unit can help to control pain, strengthen muscle, and decrease swelling. Its primary role is in the treatment of pain. It is thought to work by decreasing the effectiveness of nerves responsible for delivering pain signals. Think of pain as the volume on your stereo. A TENS unit turns down the pain volume. An uncomfortably loud squawk is changed to a gentle chirp. Electrical energy also can be used to transport medications across the skin into the deeper tissues of the knee in a process called iontophoresis. For example, a physical therapist may apply dexamethasone cream over a knee and, using an iontophoresis unit with electrodes applied to the skin, transfer the healing medication into deeper tissues without the use of a painful injection. Medications that can be driven across the skin using iontophoresis include aspirin-like medications, certain cortisone preparations, and Novocain-type drugs.

These techniques are not only used for the control of pain, swelling, and spasm, but also can be used to break up calcium deposits. In a technique called neuromuscular electrical stimulation (NMES), electricity can be used to strengthen or "re-educate" muscles. In essence, the electrical shock causes the muscle to contract. I know what you're thinking: "I could get rock-hard six-pack abs while watching *Walker, Texas Ranger* reruns." Not so fast. No one can see your abs unless you first get rid of the overlying gut. It's better to gain strength the old-fashioned way—earn it. During a workout, you lose weight and strengthen your core. Besides, electrotherapies such as TENS, galvanic stimulation, and interferential current units should be used only under the care of a trained physical therapist, as there can be major complications. Unless your therapist recommends it, back away from the electrodes, and get thee to the gym.

ULTRASOUND THERAPY

Sound energy can also be used in the treatment of arthritis. Ultrasound can penetrate through the skin and subcutaneous tissue to the deeper parts of the leg, including muscles, tendons, ligaments, and joint capsule to produce a deep heat, whose positive effects on arthritis I mentioned above. In addition, just like electricity, sound can be used to drive medication through the skin into the joint in a process called phonophoresis. An ultrasound paddle, or "head," is used to massage a mixture of ultrasound gel and medication spread over the knee joint, ideally causing the medication to penetrate into the deeper tissues. The effectiveness of iontophoresis and phonophoresis for delivering drugs into the deep tissues continues to be hotly debated by scientists.

LASER THERAPY

Low-level laser (light amplification by stimulation of emitted radiation) also can be used as therapy for arthritis. It can alter inflammation and control pain. It also has been used to heal wounds. Its biological effectiveness is still the subject of extensive research.

MASSAGE THERAPY

There's nothing like a good massage—applied mechanical energy at its finest. Use of manual therapy in the treatment of arthritis goes back thousands of years. Stroking, squeezing, and drumming of muscle can cause stimulation, with relief of spasm and pain associated with a decrease in swelling. Using so-called myofascial release and joint mobilization techniques, a physical therapist can decrease the pain of arthritis and restore motion.

Which modalities are most appropriate will depend on your therapist's assessment. The goal is to restore more function to the joint so that you can continue to work on flexibility and strength. If you have only mild arthritis, using a home-exercise program consisting of appropriate modalities, such as ice, heat, and massage, may give you significant relief. But if you have more advanced arthritis, you may need the help of a physical therapist to control pain, decrease swelling, and restore motion. Having a skilled professional apply the more sophisticated modalities we have discussed here is well worth the time and expense.

WATER PROGRAM

The therapeutic effects of water in the treatment of knee arthritis have been known for thousands of years. At the time of the pharaohs, Egyptians soaked in large wooden tubs of warm water, to which herbs and oils had been added. In other parts of the world, including the Far East, people would bask in naturally occurring mineral hot springs. The ancients enjoyed this ritual not only because of the pleasurable soak but also because of the therapeutic benefits—their joints felt better. Aquatic therapy was one of the earliest means of treating arthritis. The Greeks added minerals to warm water in the treatment of degenerative joint problems. Large communal baths utilizing natural hot springs containing carbonate minerals were used by the Romans and can be seen to this day (at Hieropolis-Pamukkale in Turkey). Both hot and cold water have been used for their therapeutic effects. In modern times we are blessed with bathtubs, hot tubs, pools, and an abundant supply of water.

Aquatic or hydrotherapy can deliver both mechanical and thermal energy directly to the skin, resulting in complex neurologic and vascular changes to the underlying tissues. Subsequent beneficial metabolic changes may occur, leading to healing. Warm, soothing water produces vasodilation and muscle relaxation, allowing painful joints to be moved more readily. Cold water, on the other hand, results in vasoconstriction and muscle tension, producing an invigorating alertness. The use of cold and hot water alternately—contrast therapy—leads to complex circulatory changes that may facilitate healing.

Water exerts pressure on anything that is submerged in it. When standing in neck-high water a person weighs about 10 percent of what he or she does on land. This is roughly analogous to living on the moon and amounts to a significant reduction in ground reaction force. The pressure of water against your body alters your circulation. The water supports and soothes the knees and applies a massage-like pressure to your lower legs, decreasing the fluid buildup around your ankles. For these reasons, many people with ankle swelling (edema) and knee arthritis benefit from pool therapy. Add Jacuzzi jets, which combine warm water and bubbles in a fifty/fifty mix, and you have the combined result of increased circulation and mechanical activation of nerve endings. To me, Jacuzzi is spelled B-L-I-S-S (blowing liquid is stimulating and salutary).

The benefits don't stop there. By significantly altering your circulation, water therapy improves healing—both to acute knee injury and chronic knee arthritis. Aquatic therapy alters the immune response. The delivery of white blood cells is increased to the arthritic knee. With increased blood flow, more oxygen is delivered to diseased tissue. The warm water also may cause your body to release endorphins—natural internal opiates that act as pain relievers and mood elevators. Your muscles relax in the presence of warm water, lowering the amount of stress on your knee joints. Water brings about changes in your mental state; you become relaxed and your stress level decreases. The effects of water therapy can last for hours after you leave the tub. Aquatic therapy in a heated pool is particularly suitable for the treatment of knee arthritis. The warm pressure effect of water decreases the pain. This enables the performance of flexibility and strengthening exercises that could not be performed on a land program. The resistance of water makes possible progressive strengthening. A unique characteristic of water is that the harder you push against it, the more it resists. This is ideal for treatment of chronically deconditioned joints and muscles of the leg. Furthermore, the water un-weights the joint because of buoyancy and allows pain-free water walking. With the help of an aquatic physical therapist, you can learn flies, scissor kicks, bicycle spins, marching, bouncing, lunges, and all manner of flexibility exercises that would be poorly tolerated on land.

Many of my patients are afraid of the water since they have never learned to swim. I tell them that the pools that are accessible in our area have protected shallow areas and are non-swimmer-friendly. Many therapists also have their patients use flotation devices for safety. Most pool therapy programs insist that their patients use footwear. This helps to prevent slipping and falling and decreases the possibility of fungal foot infections (athlete's foot). Since water can have profound effects on circulation, you should get a doctor's okay before starting an aquatic program. It is also a good idea to start a pool program under the guidance of a pool therapist. This is important from a safety standpoint but also because a skilled therapist will both assess your knee arthritis and help set up a tailor-made program for your needs.

Physical therapy is just one flanking maneuver used in the battle against knee arthritis. An old saying goes, "Give a man a fish and you feed him for a day. Teach a man to fish and you feed him for a lifetime." Physical therapy is like teaching you to fish. It will give you the guidance and the know-how that enable you to manage the symptoms of your arthritis on your own. Along with the biomechanical treatments we discussed in the previous chapter (and in some cases with the help of medicines your doctor recommends, which I will discuss in the next chapter), physical therapy literally helps to get you back on your feet again.

CHAPTER 5

PHARMACEUTICAL TREATMENT OF KNEE ARTHRITIS

I am a medical doctor specializing in orthopedic surgery. Orthopedics is the branch of medicine that deals in disorders of the musculoskeletal system—bones, joints, muscles, and tendons. The treatments that I prescribe include medication, surgery, or physical interventions that are based on rigorous scientific study and are validated by our state and federal governments, which issue licenses based on qualifications and certifications carefully delineated and enforced by law. This is not a putdown to homeopaths or practitioners of other branches of alternative medicine, but it is a warning. There is a word used to describe a doctor who prescribes placebo (ineffective medicine) drugs or procedures that he or she knows are fraudulent: a quack. A cynic might add that a placebo is a cost-effective and safe cure for the healthy neurotic. In my experience there may be a grain of truth to this.

A placebo is a sham treatment. It cannot be shown scientifically to improve the health of the patient. Nevertheless, placebos can be used to good effect in the hands of an expert. This is because many physical conditions have a psychological overlay. Remember the Cowardly Lion after he saved Dorothy from the Wicked Witch of the West? He asked the Wizard of Oz for courage, and a medal was pinned on his chest. The Lion already had proven his courage, and the medal was a placebo. A placebo can reinforce and direct the "power of positive thinking," resulting in positive and real physiological changes. But placebos should be used only as part of a multipronged and scientifically based approach to treatment.

At this point you may be wondering what all this talk of placebos has to do with the pharmaceutical treatment of arthritis. The use of medication in the treatment of disease may be fraught with controversy. According to Mark Twain, the British prime minister Benjamin Disraeli once said, "There are three kinds of lies: lies, damned lies, and statistics." Many of the studies that shape treatments used by mainstream, outcome-based medicine are based on statistical analysis. My point here is not to attack scientific methodology—I order disease-altering medication every day. The decision to prescribe a given medication involves a judgment call. Doctors have been trained to assess and diagnose your condition. Your doctor prescribes a pharmaceutical based on the drug's scientifically demonstrated efficacy and his or her familiarity with its effectiveness.

All of the medicines I discuss in this chapter are widely used by orthopedic surgeons. I use them because I have studied the research on their effectiveness and found it sufficiently compelling. Where I have been able to verify that effectiveness clinically, I continue to use them. But not all treatments work for all patients, and not all orthopedic surgeons will agree on the effectiveness of all these drugs. This will always be the case, and it is part of the reason why a multipronged approach is so important. Reasonable people may disagree in areas that are controversial.

GLUCOSAMINE AND CHONDROITIN SULFATE

I first heard about glucosamine and chondroitin sulfate (GC) as a treatment for knee arthritis about twenty years ago. A close physician friend and patient of mine had been taking it successfully for his knee arthritis. For treatment of a badly displaced bucket-handle tear of the medial meniscus, I performed knee arthroscopy on him. At the time of surgery I documented bone-on-bone arthritis of the medial compartment with an ACL-deficient knee. He was also an athlete who enjoyed rowing and skiing, although he avoided running. He kept his weight down by eating a well-balanced diet and exercising daily to maintain knee strength and flexibility. He started GC after the surgery and said his knee never bothered him. Since that time, I've suggested this over-the-counter supplement to thousands of patients with positive results. Approximately 60 percent of my patients say it helps. Many others believe that it gives them more relief than NSAIDs. Not one has ever complained of significant negative side effects to the medication.

Is GC a snake oil or the real deal? In *The Arthritis Cure (Revised Edition)*, Jason Theodosakis, MD, vigorously defended the therapeutic efficacy of GC, using studies that were available at that time. He argued that the GC combination should be "pure" and of adequate concentration: 1500 mg of glucosamine and 1200 mg of chondroitin sulfate. His arguments were persuasive and presented in an attractive written format. Since Dr. Theodosakis's book was published, further studies of GC's efficacy have been published. An article in the *New England Journal of Medicine* in 2006 suggested that GC might not be significantly more effective than placebo. The GAIT (GC Arthritis Intervention Trial) study performed by the National Institutes of Health in 2010 also suggested that patients taking GC had similar outcomes to those who took Celebrex or placebo. I'm not sure what the study tells us about Celebrex.

But before you cry "fraud" or "quack," quietly and reasonably examine the evidence. Many excellent studies performed in both Europe and North America have validated the effectiveness of GC. Other studies have suggested it is worthless. Strong emotional opinions have come from both sides, many with vested interests. For approximately thirty-five dollars you can buy a two-month supply of GC. That amount of money will buy you approximately seven Celebrex tablets. Many patients with arthritis will use two Celebrex tablets per day, although it has never been demonstrated to work better than simple aspirin in treatment of knee arthritis. I can purchase aspirin for less than one penny a tablet at the grocery store. You may not be surprised that the use of Celebrex for the treatment of arthritis is strongly advocated by its maker (witness the commercials on TV).

Despite the discrepancy in expert opinion, you should be aware that many practitioners continue to use GC as a safe, economic, and possibly effective treatment of knee arthritis. The continued use of this medication is supported by many scientific studies. I've seen many patients start the medication and do well while others show no response, although none, to my knowledge, have been harmed. In my hands, GC is never used as the sole treatment of arthritis but is used in conjunction with an integrated approach (i.e., diet, exercise, NSAIDs, and good, healthy life choices). In short, the use of GC does not pose an ethical dilemma to me. I wouldn't be surprised if within five years a better and stronger type of GC were released that put an end to the scientific confusion. Give me a better, safer treatment for arthritis, and I'll use it. For now, I'll use the best and safest medicines available.

NSAIDS (NONSTEROIDAL ANTI-INFLAMMATORY DRUGS)

Inflammation is part of the healing response to tissue that has been injured or has become diseased. This response involves white blood cells (acting as microscopic warriors fighting disease) and blood vessels, which provide the vascular roads by which these cells can reach the war zone (area of injury or disease). There are five signs of inflammation described in Latin: *calor* (heat), *rubor* (redness), *tumor* (swelling), *dolor* (pain), and *functio laesa* (loss of function). An anti-inflammatory drug (like ibuprofen) treats all the signs of inflammation. Some drugs, such as Tylenol (acetaminophen), are analgesics, or pain relievers, and not anti-inflammatory drugs. Although they can treat the pain of arthritis, they do not alter the fundamental cause of the problem, which is inflammation.

Anti-inflammatory drugs are divided into two categories: those that contain steroids and those that do not. I will discuss the steroidal drug cortisone later. NSAID is a common acronym that stands for non-steroidal anti-inflammatory drug. These are safer, although less potent, than steroids in the treatment of inflammation. The NSAIDs are often the first line of defense against arthritis. The prototypical NSAID is aspirin, or acetylsalicylic acid. It is an ancient "miracle" drug. Hippocrates, the father of Western medicine, who lived around 400 BC, used salicylic tea in the treatment of fevers and pain. Salicylate is an extract of willow bark. The Egyptian pharaohs mentioned the use of willow as a medicine in their papyri. Lewis and Clark, in their famous exploration of the American West, used willow bark tea to treat fever. Native American healers used willow leaves and bark as part of their treatment for headaches, pain, and fevers. In around 1829, Henri Leroux, a French pharmacist, isolated salicin from willow bark. In 1897, Felix Hoffman synthetically created acetylsalicylic acid (ASA). Modern aspirin was introduced and marketed by Bayer around the turn of the twentieth century. This wonder drug is used for control of pain, headaches, and fever. Because it decreases the stickiness of platelets, resulting in thinning of the blood, it is used to treat cardiovascular disease. It is used for the treatment and prevention of blood clots and may even help in the prevention of cancer of the colon. And—you guessed it—it is also used in the treatment of arthritis. All the other more than one hundred NSAIDs on the market were created after the discovery of aspirin. The newest additions to the family of NSAIDs are called the Cox-2 inhibitors. You may recognize their names—Celebrex, Bextra, and Vioxx. The FDA removed the last two from the market because of dangerous cardiovascular side effects. Celebrex remains as an expensive prescription drug with specific medical indications.

The most popular NSAID today is ibuprofen. You've seen it in the store as generic ibuprofen or brand name Advil, Nuprin, or Motrin. Another popular NSAID is naproxen—also known as brand name Aleve or Naprosyn. These two medications can be purchased over the counter (OTC). Most of the other NSAIDs require a doctor's prescription—for a reason. There are many side effects to this class of drugs, including stomach upset, peptic ulcers, high blood pressure, asthma, easy bruising, bleeding, kidney failure, and severe allergic reaction. When these medications are taken properly they can be very effective and relatively safe. But consider yourself warned—don't take even over-the-counter NSAIDs for long periods of time. The *American Journal of Medicine* stated in 1998, "At least 16,500 NSAID related deaths occur each year among arthritis patients alone."

So how do you minimize the dangerous side effects of NSAIDs? Don't take them regularly for more than two weeks. If your knee is not bothering you, don't take medication. If you notice indigestion or rectal bleeding, stop the drug immediately and call your doctor. Some physicians have patients take NSAIDs with Cytotec or Tums to protect against GI upset and ulcers. Take the medication with a bite of food. Make sure to drink eight glasses of water daily to protect your kidneys. Don't smoke and use alcohol when taking NSAIDs. Don't ever mix one NSAID with a different one. Don't take them if you're on any blood-thinning medication like Plavix, aspirin, or Coumadin. Be careful—you don't want to be a statistic.

Many of my patients ask me about Celebrex (celecoxib). It is a selective Cox-2 inhibitor used in the treatment of arthritis. It was initially introduced as a safer alternative to standard NSAIDs that caused fewer ulcers. However, it has been shown to be associated with occasional serious cardiovascular problems, including elevation of blood pressure, heart attacks, and strokes. It does not "thin" the blood, as standard NSAIDs do, and can therefore be used at the same time as the blood thinner Coumadin. In my opinion, Celebrex is rarely indicated because of its potential danger and expense.

Like all the treatments described here, NSAIDs should not be used alone in the treatment of arthritis but as one valuable weapon among many in the attack against arthritis.

ACETAMINOPHEN

Although not classified as an NSAID, acetaminophen, or Tylenol, has been used in the treatment of arthritis pain since the 1950s. Outside of North America, it is called paracetamol. Tylenol does have pain-relieving, fever-breaking, and mild anti-inflammatory properties. Approximately one-third of people with arthritis who take acetaminophen will notice some relief of pain.

In 2011 the FDA issued a warning regarding the safety of Tylenol. They limited the amount of acetaminophen in each tablet to 325 mg. You may recall that Tylenol Extra Strength used to be 500 mg per tablet. The FDA stated that this was too much acetaminophen and posed a health risk. They warned of possible severe liver damage and allergic reactions. From 1998 to 2003, acetaminophen was the leading cause of acute liver failure in the United States, according to FDA data. A 2013 episode of *This American Life* ("Use Only as Directed") claimed that acetaminophen kills more people than any other over-the-counter medication. Commonly, drug manufacturers combine other drugs with Tylenol, including caffeine, aspirin, butalbital, codeine, hydrocodone, oxycodone, pentazocine, and tramadol. The FDA suggests that patients not exceed 4 g per day of acetaminophen. Ingesting other liver-toxic medications, such as alcohol, worsens the possible toxic effect of Tylenol. What do many people use for treating a hangover? Tylenol! This is big mistake that can have disastrous consequences. I rarely suggest using acetaminophen for the treatment of knee arthritis.

OPIOIDS

Often, knee arthritis results in chronic pain. If the pain is not controlled by other medications, such as OTC pain relievers and NSAIDs, your physician may prescribe narcotic or opioid medications. Although arthritis is generally a chronic condition, it may be made worse—for a variety of reasons—for short periods (exacerbation) or even permanently (aggravation). If the pain is severe, opioids are indicated, usually for a short period of time, so that other treatment modalities may be started.

The word narcotic is derived from an ancient Greek verb meaning "to become numb." In the United States, the word is associated with opioids like morphine and its opium-derived family members. (The word opiate should be used precisely to refer to the natural alkaloids found in the opium poppy resin.) Like aspirin, the effects of opium have been appreciated for thousands of years. The ancient Sumerian, Egyptian, and Greeks all used it for pain relief. Very little has changed. Modern opioids are still used as some of the most effective pain relievers available. The ancient drug morphine remains the gold standard by which all other major pain relievers are measured. But like any fine two-edged sword, it has sharp edges that, if not carefully controlled, can cause great damage to the user. Too much may cause an overdose and death. If used for a lengthy period of time and then stopped suddenly, withdrawal symptoms may occur. Prolonged and improper use of the drug may result in tolerance and addiction—both psychological and physical. Even when used properly it has powerful adverse effects, which include nausea, vomiting, and constipation. All of the opioids share the same negative side effects as morphine. Despite their adverse effects, because of their efficacy and euphoric side effects they remain some of the most abused drugs known, exceeded only by another ancient but legal drug—alcohol.

If function can be restored to an arthritic patient in chronic, disabling pain with the use of opioids, then it is reasonable to prescribe them. The caveat is that the patient must be carefully monitored for adverse side effects, including progressive habituation to the drug. A patient in chronic pain is substantially different from the illicit drug abuser who is looking for a high. Rather than causing impairment, proper use of opiates as effective pain relievers may restore functionality to someone disabled with arthritis. Physical dependence and opiate tolerance may occur in the older arthritic but, in my opinion, do not lead to drug abuse. On rare occasions I will draw up a "pain contract" with patients when prescribing opiates for chronic pain. This arrangement can give them their lives back. I have yet to see an octogenarian "break bad."

Skeptics might retort, "You're just covering the symptoms of arthritis instead of curing it" with the use of narcotics. By a "cure," such critics usually mean surgical intervention and total knee replacement (TKR). But may I respectfully ask, since when is a TKR a cure? While I have advanced training in joint replacement and have performed well over a thousand of these operations, I regard it as a salvage procedure that gives fair to good results at best and is indicated only when non-operative conservative measures have failed to provide relief. Although the operation may improve the pain and function of someone with end-stage arthritis, the replacement cannot be compared to a normal knee. Substituting the cartilage with plastic and metal removes the biologic surface of the knee. The way the knee moves biomechanically is substantially changed after replacement. Nerves are invariably cut during the surgery, resulting in numbness over the outer aspect of the knee. Because some of the restraining ligaments are released during the procedure, the patient is often left with mild to moderate instability. How many patients following TKR can descend a stairway without using the railing? How many can run? The surgery is major and associated with risks and complications, including blood clots, infection, chronic leg swelling, instability, loosening of the prosthesis, loss of motion, nerve damage resulting in chronic leg weakness and numbness, persistent knee pain, hospital-acquired infections, amputation, and anesthesia death. And the cost is up to fifty thousand dollars after everyone is paid. Wow! It makes you want to rush out and have one done—not! And yet desperate people take desperate measures. When the knee pain from arthritis can no longer be tolerated, then it is reasonable to proceed with this major operation. But let us remember George Bernard Shaw's warning that doctors make more money when they operate than when they don't.

CORTISONE

I mentioned above that anti-inflammatory drugs could be steroidal or non-steroidal. Steroids include complex compounds naturally produced in your body. You've heard of testosterone and estrogen. They are steroids. But there are other types of steroids that have anti-inflammatory properties. Synthetic corticosteroids, like prednisone and cortisone, are the most powerful anti-inflammatory drugs available and can be used in the treatment of arthritis with success. However, they have troubling and sometimes frightening side effects when taken orally or given intravenously, including fluid retention, elevated blood sugar (especially in the presence of diabetes), osteoporosis, decreased immunity, a type of aggressive hip arthritis called avascular necrosis of the femoral head, bruising and thinning of the skin, cataracts, and occasionally psychotic behavior. These potent drugs can be life-saving, but should be used with caution. Since arthritis can have an inflammatory element, cortisone can be very effective in its treatment. If NSAIDs and OTC medications have not helped alleviate your knee arthritis pain, then the next step may be a cortisone shot. Your doctor will decide.

The effects of cortisone are local—limited to where the shot is given—rather than systemic. Thus, the common side effects of other steroids, like prednisone, are not seen. A cortisone injection to the knee should be almost pain-free. The skin is first prepared with an antiseptic such as Betadine or alcohol. A topical anesthetic aerosol called ethyl chloride, which temporarily "freezes" the skin, is then applied to take away the pain of the needle. The cortisone is injected with lidocaine—an anesthetic to remove the pain caused by corticosteroid crystals. Most patients note almost instantaneous relief of arthritic pain following the injection. I instruct my patients to take it easy on the knee for two to three days to allow the cortisone to absorb into the tissues. The knee should be iced for twenty minutes the day of the injection. The great majority of patients derive from six to twelve weeks of knee pain relief following a cortisone injection. The shot does not just "cover" the pain; it attacks the root cause—inflammation. This allows you to work on flexibility and strength, which in the long term will decrease the symptoms of knee arthritis. Corticosteroid injections may be associated with some minor complications. A painful short-lived "cortisone flare" may occur at the site of the injection, usually subsiding after one or two days with ice and NSAIDs. If the corticosteroid penetrates the subcutaneous tissue, then "blanching" of the skin may occur. The benefits of the cortisone outweigh its risks, in my experience.

VISCOSUPPLEMENTATION: HYALURONIC ACID

As we discussed in the section on the anatomy of the knee, one of the major characteristics of osteoarthritis is a loss of hyaluronic acid (a major component of the synovial fluid). Hyaluronic acid (HA) traps water for the purpose of lubricating the knee joint and so guarantees cartilage surfaces that are more slippery. As arthritis progresses, the amount and quality of hyaluronic acid changes, resulting in increased friction during motion. This produces inflammation—heat, swelling, and stiffness associated with pain and loss of function. In an attempt to restore a slippery cushion in the knee, injectable viscous preparations of HA, generically called viscosupplementation (VS), are used.

Proponents of HA supplementation claim that it acts as a lubricant and shock absorber with possible anti-inflammatory effects. One advocate is the FDA, which has approved it for the treatment of osteoarthritis of the knee. It has been used in Europe for the treatment of knee arthritis since the 1980s. To my knowledge, there are now five kinds available in the United States: Hyalgen, Orthovisc, Supartz, Synvisc, and Euflexxa. They are administered in a series of injections given one week apart. Recently, two others have been introduced that are delivered in one injection only—Synvisc 1 and Gel 1. A significant body of scientific evidence supports the use of VS in the treatment of knee arthritis. In 2013, however, the American Academy of Orthopedic Surgeons stated strongly in its Clinical Practice Guidelines, "We cannot recommend using hyaluronic acid for patients with symptomatic osteoarthritis of the knee."

As usual, it's a matter of whom to believe. Many studies suggest that knee pain in 80 percent of patients will diminish for approximately six months to one year after the injections. It has been my clinical experience that HA does indeed help relieve arthritic knee symptoms. After using several types of HA, I began using a formulation made from non-animal/non-avian protein. It is not unusual to see a patient obtain two to three years of pain relief after a series of three injections. To my knowledge, none of my patients has been made worse by the injections.

HA has a very definite role in the treatment of knee arthritis, but like the other treatments discussed in this section, it should be used as one weapon among many to combat knee arthritis. Positive results include decreased swelling, improved motion, and better function with less pain. Most people experience minimal discomfort during the injection and are able to return to their normal activities without significant problems. Although not recommended, I've even had patients attend dances the evening after the injection.

I have seen several reactions, such as painful redness and swelling, when using an HA preparation derived from chicken protein. The injections are approved by Medicare and most insurance companies and can be repeated every six months as needed. I teach my patients that using HA is like hitting foul balls—you can continue ninety-nine times. I have many patients who have used HA successfully every six-to-twelve-months for well over five years, successfully avoiding total knee replacement. Unfortunately, HA doesn't work for everyone, but in the majority of patients, it offers significant relief.

PART THREE

AN ARTHRITIS-FREE LIFESTYLE—
MAINTAINING YOUR MOBILITY

CHAPTER 6

EATING TO BE ARTHRITIS-FREE

So far we have looked at the problem of arthritis and how to fix it. I have repeatedly used cars as a metaphor. In many ways, our bodies are like cars. When properly kept, your vehicle can last for years. In order to ensure long life, however, we must have at least some idea of how they work and must repair them when needed. An old proverb says, "A stitch in time saves nine." That's maintenance. If we take good care of things every day and not just when they're broken, chances are they won't break in the first place. Regular oil changes, gasket replacements, cleaning—these are all ways we take care of our cars. Maintenance of the human body means living a healthy lifestyle— eating well, staying active, getting enough sleep, and so on.

In the last part of this book I am going to discuss how maintenance is the most important thing you can do to keep the symptoms of knee arthritis at bay. In this chapter I'll focus on the importance of diet. Then, in chapter seven, we'll look at ways you can live a physically active lifestyle. Finally, in the last chapter we'll consider how all the little lifestyle choices we make every single day contribute to the health of our knees.

For those who suffer from mild arthritis, it may be enough to make alterations to your lifestyle to get yourself on the road to healthier knees. Patients suffering from more advanced arthritis may have to do some remedial work before benefiting fully from the recommendations in this final part of the book. That's what the preceding three chapters are about. With the help of the treatments there, you'll be able to clean the slate, so to speak—to correct as much of the damage as possible caused by unhealthy living and the disease that results from it. Once you've lost weight and brought the debilitating symptoms of arthritis, like pain and inflammation, under control, you'll be in a position to start rebuilding your life. It is going to require some dedication and increased awareness on your part. Lots of old habits will have to be broken. But if you take seriously the recommendations I provide here, I can guarantee that your knees will work and feel better.

REASONS TO WATCH WHAT YOU EAT

In chapter three we talked about diets. What we meant there were programs designed specifically to help you lose weight. Excessive weight is a major cause of knee osteoarthritis, and getting your weight down to a healthy level is the single most important thing you can do to mitigate arthritis symptoms. But weight loss is only a fix. When you fix your car it's not a one-time deal, something you never have to worry about again. It's the same with your physical health. Once you get your body to a healthy place, you need to take daily steps to maintain it there. So when I talk about diet in this chapter, I am talking not about a weight-loss strategy but about a regular and sustainable way of eating (that cannot be isolated from a way of living, which we will discuss in the next two chapters) that *keeps* the weight from coming back. In a minute we'll look at the rudiments of healthy eating (nutrition), and then we'll go on to see that a healthy diet can take many different forms—just as an unhealthy diet can. My objective will be to give you the resources to understand what is and what is not healthy and with that understanding to make informed decisions about how you eat. But first, let's look at a few reasons why managing your diet is a good idea. These are meant to be motivators.

There are many reasons to watch what you eat. If your dog was starting to gain unhealthy weight, you'd cut back on his Ken-L rations. But self-discipline, it seems, is the most difficult discipline to enforce. A hungry person seldom examines what he is eating in the rush to wish fulfillment. Much of my time in the office is spent encouraging people to eat wisely. Next time you find yourself reaching for that unhealthy comfort food, think about the following advantages to eating well.

1. You will become lean. By eating less and exercising more, you will notice increased energy. Your knees will ache less as flexibility and strength return, allowing you to exercise more.

2. You will be eating good, nutritious food yet will lose weight, putting less stress on your knees. Your feeling of well-being will improve. Your thinking will become clearer as you change your diet from one full of bad carbohydrates to one with healthy carbs, like spinach, beet greens, broccoli, and cauliflower—good veggies rich in vitamins A, B, C, D, E, and K.

3. As you reset your hunger thermostat, you'll enjoy eating more. If you are conscious of the food you eat, you'll eat more slowly, enjoying each bite instead of thoughtlessly wolfing down a box of warm, greasy sugar doughnuts or a bag of potato chips.

4. As you eat healthier foods with fewer calories, your sleep cycles will improve. Not only will you retire at night without that full feeling, but also—because you were more energetic during the day—you will nod off when your head hits the pillow and sleep soundly.

5. Your overall health will improve. Your knee arthritis will be less symptomatic. You will be less prone to develop many of the degenerative diseases that accompany advancing age, such as diabetes, heart disease, osteoporosis, and cancer. You will add life to your years and not just years to your life, truly enjoying the "golden years."

NUTRITION: THE BUILDING BLOCKS OF A HEALTHY DIET

Ah, food—the fuel of life. In America, "breadbasket of the world," we've been blessed with an over-abundance of food. But while guaranteeing our food supply, this blessing is mixed. What we've gained in quantity, we've sacrificed in quality. We need to begin with an understanding of why some foods are healthy and others are not. The science of nutrition looks at the health value (the quality) of food. The elements in food that contribute to its value to our bodies are called nutrients, and they are conventionally divided into two groups: macronutrients and micronutrients.

Macro means "big" in Greek, and the macronutrients are the big three elements of food: carbohydrates, protein, and fat. Together, they provide the fuel that is converted to energy when digested. It's much the same as when we put wood into a stove, generating heat to boil water. The energy runs the complex machine that is our body. Energy is measured in calories. The macronutrient with the most calories is fat, at nine calories per gram. Protein and carbohydrates each have four calories per gram. It makes sense to store excess fuel in the body as fat rather than carbohydrates or protein, as fat holds more potential energy by weight.

Carbohydrates, or carbs, are our main form of fuel, essential and readily used by the body's cells in the form of glucose. Without glucose you would seize and then die. The heart and brain depend on it as their major source of energy. Glucose is stored in both muscle and the liver for quick access to energy (like pocket money, easy to get to), rather than at some distant fat storage site (like money in the bank, a hassle to get to). Some carbs, in the form of fiber, are not digested and pass through our intestines, acting like millions of little squeegees keeping our gut clean and healthy. Foods rich in carbohydrates include starchy foods (potatoes, pasta, rice, grain, bread, pizza, bagels, doughnuts, and whoopee pies—a New England favorite), vegetables, and fruit.

Proteins are a necessary part of muscle, helping to build, maintain, and repair it. They are also indispensable to the formation of hormones and all kinds of tissue in your body. Foods rich in protein include meat, seafood, soy and dairy products, eggs, nuts, and beans.

Fat is more than just the storage form of fuel. It works well as a cushion, protecting important organs from damage, including our hearts, intestines, and kidneys. It allows for comfort during sitting. Fat is also a very important part of cell walls. The brain is composed of around 60 percent fat. It is also essential in the absorption of certain important vitamins—A, D, E, and K. Fat has been unfairly maligned as the cause of the obesity epidemic. But without dietary fat, we would eventually die.

Micronutrients are other essential nutrients needed only in very small amounts. They include vitamins, minerals, and essential amino acids. Without certain vitamins, life would be short. Some vitamins dissolve in water (water-soluble vitamins). These are not stored in the body as they are washed out in your urine and must be replaced every day. The most famous may be vitamin C, which is found in fresh fruit and vegetables. Then there is the vitamin B complex, which includes B3, B6, B12, and folic acid. The other group of vitamins dissolves in fat (fat-soluble) and includes vitamins A, D, E, and K.

They need to be dissolved in fat before they can be used by the body and can be stored in the liver, meaning that you do not need to replace them daily.

We need a lot of certain minerals. These are called macrominerals and include calcium, phosphorous, potassium, sodium, and chloride. Other minerals are needed only in small amounts. These are called—you guessed it— microminerals and include iron, zinc, copper, selenium, and iodine. These are found in many common foods naturally and are often added to others. Some organic compounds, including amino acids, are also required to carry out basic life functions like growth and repair. Many of these building blocks of life, the essential amino acids, can only be provided by our diet.

Without micronutrients, horrible and predictable diseases of deficiency occur. Without enough vitamin C, you'll get scurvy. Insufficient folic acid can result in birth defects, including spina bifida. Take out the vitamin D, and rickets and osteomalacia will be the result. Vitamin D, you may remember, is also essential to the health of our bones. To be useful, it must be converted to its active form by exposure to sunlight. For this reason, in some northern states it may be necessary to take a vitamin D supplement in the wintertime to make sure you're getting enough. Vitamin A deficiency leads to poor vision. Without iron you get anemia. The list goes on. The good news is that a healthy diet automatically contains most of these micronutrients. Eat your veggies!

Another nutritional concept we need to understand before we talk about food is the glycemic index. As I mentioned briefly when talking about carbohydrates, glucose ("blood sugar") is necessary to maintain life-providing energy to our organ systems—liver, brain, muscles, etc. With a low-circulating glucose comes weakness, confusion, and ultimately seizures and death. Your body carefully monitors the amount of circulating blood glucose. If your blood sugar increases, insulin is secreted by the pancreas to decrease the glucose level by causing it to be absorbed into the cells of your body. If the glucose is too low, muscle can be broken down into glucose. Low glucose also triggers hunger pangs. Certain foods cause the glucose to shoot sky-high. We've all seen what happens when a six-year-old eats a box of jujubes—an Energizer Bunny bouncing off the walls on a sugar high. Other foods with low sugar content do not significantly elevate glucose at all—a glass of whole milk, for example.

There is a way to measure the effect of food on your blood glucose. It's called the glycemic index (GI). Eating pure glucose gives a GI of 100. Foods with a high GI are digested and absorbed into the bloodstream quickly. Foods with a low GI are digested and absorbed slowly. High-GI foods include the following: corn chips, white bread, doughnuts, bagels, and candy. Low GI foods include grapefruit, beans, berries, oatmeal, and many vegetables. Most other food falls in the middle somewhere and include sweet corn, pizza, whole wheat, and plain vanilla ice cream.

If you eat too many foods that have a high GI on a regular basis, you run the risk of having consistently high blood glucose, which taxes your pancreas as it struggles to produce more insulin. By regularly packing away high-GI food, repetitive sugar spikes can result in pancreatic stress and ultimately failure. Under these circumstances, insulin levels are chronically high and the cells of the body resist its influence. They are like parents surrounded by a teenager constantly playing high-energy rock—they turn down the volume or use earplugs. Chronically elevated blood glucose and its aftermath can result in the so-called metabolic syndrome. In short, the metabolic syndrome consists of five features: (1) elevated gut fat ("beer belly" or "inner tube"); (2) high triglycerides; (3) low "good" cholesterol (HDL); (4) high blood pressure; and (5) elevated fasting blood sugar (pre-diabetes and type 2 diabetes). The metabolic syndrome drastically increases the possibility of stroke, heart disease, and diabetes and can lead to or worsen knee arthritis. In other words, you don't want the metabolic syndrome.

So what's the takeaway? Your diet should be composed of mostly low or moderate GI foods that are nutrient-rich. Fiber is good because it decreases the absorption of sugar. Avoid sugar.

THE WAY WE EAT, OR PYRAMIDS AREN'T ONLY IN EGYPT

In 1992 the United States Department of Agriculture introduced the "official" food pyramid. A pyramid is built from the base up and is wider at the bottom. In the USDA's figurative one, food groups lying at the bottom of the pyramid are to be eaten in greater quantities than those at the top. The bottom layer of the pyramid consists of carbohydrate-rich foods like pasta, rice, grain, cereal, and bread. The layer above that, eaten in smaller quantities, is vegetables and fruits. The next level is milk products, such as cheese and yogurt, as well as protein, including meat, fish, and eggs. The food group at the top of the pyramid, eaten sparingly, includes fats, oils, and sweets. When I first looked at the pyramid, I thought, "Makes sense." The common acceptance of this pyramid as gospel has led to an increase in obesity over the last twenty years.

The food industry jumped on the bandwagon with both feet. That jump has been nothing but trouble for both of your knees. A stroll through your local supermarket will show you the effect it has had. The "low-fat" or "fat-free" label is found on virtually every box of refined food on the shelves. Buyer beware! "Low-fat," as you now know, does not mean low calories. Some of these refined foods are not only very caloric but are chock-full of chemicals that I can't even pronounce and certainly don't want to eat. Then there are the "sugar-free" prepared foods. Although sugar, in any significant quantity, is bad for you, sugar replacements may be even worse. Several of them have been implicated in causing cancer. If you're interested in the way we eat in America, I strongly suggest you read Michael Pollan's book *In Defense of Food*. The author unravels, in a common-sense way, the complex evolution of industrialized food and concludes that we need to get back to basics—that is, eat simple, whole foods, preferably locally grown. His solution is so simple even I can understand it: "Eat food. Not too much. Mostly plants."

What is remarkable is that many so-called traditional cultures have been nutritionally healthy, even as their diets diverge widely from one another. Consider the Masai people of Kenya. They survive on a protein-dense diet consisting of a mixture of milk and blood (Atkins diet to the extreme), augmented by starch and carbohydrates. They are, as a group, lean and athletic, capable of effortlessly walking great distances and almost completely free of arthritis. They live in a very hostile environment—the Great Rift Valley—and if they survive early childhood, they generally thrive as adults. They eat no processed food, have low body weights, get plenty of exercise, and have almost no knee arthritis.

Okinawans, to take another example, maintain good health into great age. They eat a diet dense with green and yellow vegetables (sweet potatoes), tofu, fish, and pork. They eat virtually no eggs or milk products. They practice a tradition that, roughly translated, states, "Eat until you are 80 percent full." In addition, they get plenty of exercise. What have we here? Homegrown food, no processed or canned food, thin and physically active people, and very little knee arthritis.

Then there are the Sardinians. Their diet is simple and homegrown. It is rich in milk and cheese. A snack of red wine, sheep's cheese, and olives is not unusual. A common toast is, "May you live to be a hundred." And many do. They eat simple carbohydrates—native vegetables, minestrone, bread— and proportionately large quantities of olive oil. Their meat delicacy is suckling pig. This diet is one of the eating traditions that gave rise to the term "Mediterranean diet." It is high in fiber (healthy leafy vegetables), high in protein (including cheese and meat), contains healthy fat (in the form of olive oil), with moderate amounts of red wine. What is the secret to their longevity? Probably many things, including genetics, hard physical and purposeful work, a tight-knit community that respects age and accomplishment, a mild climate, good food, and exercise. Sardinians are slender walkers who enjoy "slow food" and have hardly any knee arthritis.

The case of the Inuit is also instructive. These Arctic dwellers live in one of the harshest climates on earth and thrive. Their diet, to anyone who has ever looked at the food pyramid, seems like a recipe for disaster. The frozen tundra is devoid of plant life for most of the year. Consequently, the Inuit derive nearly all of their calories from fat and protein. Their principal food sources include seal, walrus, whale, caribou, and fish. Over 50 percent of their caloric intake is from fat. Thirty to forty percent of their calories come from protein. The Inuit have claimed that their diet is perfect, giving them energy and keeping them warm during the cold, long winters. They live an active physical lifestyle while hunting and simply surviving in an uncompromising environment. They have almost no knee arthritis. Supporting the viability of such a diet is the case of celebrated Minnesota dog musher Will Steger, who drove his sled from Duluth to the North Pole and in 1986 headed the first confirmed team to reach the North Pole unsupported, while subsisting on a diet of raw caribou meat and butter. Steger is five foot nine and weighs 142 pounds.

Finally, there is the "bush tucker" diet of the Australian Aborigines. Their traditional lifestyle is reasonably characterized as a hunter-gatherer type. The coming-of-age of a young man is classically ushered in by a "walkabout." The youth wanders through the bush for up to six months, following "songlines" of ancestors (reliving visions of the past). The aboriginal culture is ancient; painted rock art in the Kakadu National Park in the Outback is estimated to be sixty thousand years old. Formerly the aboriginal people would forage and hunt through the country, often traveling large distances. They ate off the land, taking what was available. Their diet was low in calories but high in nutrient value. Carbs consisted of grass, plants, roots, fruit, and nuts. Honey, in particular, was relished as a treat. Depending on whether they were in the bush or near the coast, 40 to 80 percent of their diet was from plant sources. Fat and protein came from many sources, including grubs, turtles, snakes, kangaroo, possum, fish, small freshwater crocodiles, and tree ants. They were masters of the terrain and knew where the water supply was in this arid land. They drank large quantities of pure water—by some estimates, twice what Europeans consume. They viewed certain foods as essential to good health, while other food and herbs were used in the treatment of disease. Take, for example, eucalyptus. The oil of the eucalyptus was used to treat many illnesses, including asthma and bronchitis. It has been shown to have pain-control and anti-inflammatory properties. In short, historical Aborigines walked a lot, ate a lot of low-caloric healthy food, and had almost no knee arthritis.

What conclusions can we draw from this interesting review of different cultural practices regarding diet and its relationship to knee arthritis? How can we attain a knee-healthy diet? One conclusion would be to relocate to the Masai Mara of Kenya, the Ryukyu Islands of southern Japan, an isolated island in the Mediterranean, Nunavut or Greenland, or "the Alice" in Australia's Northern Territory. Of course, you would have to become a local. For example, in the Outback you'd have to learn to play the didgeridoo and become proficient with the boomerang. In the Arctic you'd have to learn the art of building an igloo, mukluk repair, and understand the migratory patterns of polar bears. In Africa you'd need to learn how to trephine a cow and do the jump dance. There's got to be an easier way to healthy knees.

How can these diverse groups of people all have better knee health than we do? I mean, aren't we an advanced digital society? We are blessed and cursed. We exercise less and eat more of the wrong type of food, when compared to other cultures. The wrong type means food with too many calories and not enough nutrient value.

We've never had a more plentiful or diverse supply of food in the United States than now. This has occurred as a result of miraculous advances in industrial farming practices and food preservation. The use of pesticides, chemical fertilizers, and genetic engineering has allowed us to produce abundant food of poor quality. Compare the large, glossy red tomato at the supermarket with one grown in your backyard using compost as fertilizer. Which looks better? Undoubtedly, the store-bought tomato is more appealing to the eye. Which has the better flavor? Without question, the homegrown fruit tastes better. How about meat? The succulent, juicy-appearing chicken in your supermarket is often raised in a cage and force-fed a diet adulterated with antibiotics, contaminated gluten, and animal waste. After mechanized slaughter, the meat is injected with brine, immediately prior to presentation at the store, to give it a healthy and luscious appearance. Compare this with a smaller, free-range, organically fed chicken. I suggest you spend the extra money and taste the difference—chicken raised the old-fashioned way is tastier. The same rules apply to beef. Free-range, plus hormone-free, plus antibiotic-free, plus grass fed and finished equals more nutritious and better-tasting food. Remember, you are what you eat. So if you want to be healthy and thin, eat healthy and eat less.

I mentioned that the processing of food is the other industrial "miracle" that has led to the dazzling abundance on our supermarket shelves. Processing originated as a way of making possible the preservation of food during a time of plenty so it could be eaten during a time of need. The practice dates back thousands of years. In ancient days, smoking, sun drying, pickling, and salting meat and fish allowed foods to be preserved for long periods. Kippers, an ancestral food of the Scots, were the highlanders' version of processed food. Carbohydrates have also been processed for a very long time. A staple food of British sailors was hardtack—a simple mixture of flour, water, and salt that is baked in low heat, resulting in a hard and dehydrated biscuit. This resilient "tack" would last months without decomposition. It gained its nickname, "molar breakers," as a result of its extraordinary hardness. My son Anders depended on hardtack as a major food source when he crossed northern Canada in winter during a solo cross-country ski trip a few years ago. Then there's the classic kosher pickle, an outstanding example of old-school processed food—a summer vegetable preserved through fermentation. Let us not forget this most ancient form of food processing of all—the fermenting of liquids. A fermented fluid lasts a long time without degrading—and contains alcohol. This energy-rich drink is primarily valued for its most notable side effect: intoxication.

There are inarguably clear benefits associated with processing food. The food lasts longer and can be transported great distances. In addition, processing food can eliminate disease-causing bacteria. Pasteurization has saved millions of lives and prevented undue misery by removing the tuberculosis bacillus from milk. Processed food is convenient, inexpensive, readily prepared, and generally regarded as safe, if not the healthiest of choices. But there is a dark side to this scientific manipulation of food.

Enter mechanization, the large-scale industrial preparation of processed food. If it can be canned, boxed, bottled, or bagged by the food industry, and it has been. The result of this is the modern supermarket. It is a chemical cornucopia of "wannabe" food. Michael Pollan describes modern processed foods as "edible food-like substances." They are mass-produced in factories for transportation over great distances and able to be stored for months or even years. Such food is often characterized as "artificial." The smell, taste, color, and consistency are often fake, the effect of non-nutritional additives. Processing often occurs via added chemicals (stabilizers), some of which are toxic. Many food additives can make people sick and even die. Peanut oil, a common additive, can be fatal to those with a peanut allergy. Too much sodium chloride can increase blood pressure. Added sugar can precipitate or worsen diabetes. Some additives may result in an increased risk of cancer and arthritis, including that of the knee. Other chemicals may alter the state of your hormonal health, resulting in loss of sex drive (consider the frequency of Viagra and Cialis commercials on TV).

And think about how some of these prepared foods are packaged. Polycarbonate plastic bottles contain bisphenol A (BPA), an environmental estrogen. BPA is an endocrine disruptor. It has been shown to have harmful effects on lab animals and is thought by some researchers to have a similar effect on humans. Putting boiling water in plastic bottles increases dramatically the rate of leaching of BPA from the plastic. I cringe when thinking of the hundreds of gallons of water I've consumed from plastic hiking bottles over the years. Some scientists have implicated BPA as one more cause of obesity. The jury is still out as to whether BPA leads to nerve damage, endocrine dysfunction, and cancer in humans. It is, at any rate, very suspect. What about aluminum cans? Aluminum is toxic to your central nervous system and has been implicated as one of the causes of Alzheimer's disease. Here again, the connection has not been scientifically validated. I don't know about you, but I'm forgetful enough without challenging my nervous system with doses of aluminum. It took our federal government many years to establish the causal relationship between cigarette smoking and lung cancer with certainty. Any reasonable person should be concerned about the possible health hazards of how foods are packaged.

What about canned food? The inside of steel cans is often coated with plastic to protect from bacteria and metal corrosion. Aha! We've just seen that plastic leaches out BPA when exposed to heat. Add to this that industrially canned food generally has high levels of sodium. And there's more. Sulfites are often used as preservatives in canning. Sulfites include sulfur dioxide, potassium bisulfite, potassium metabisulfite, and sodium sulfide. They can cause severe allergic reactions in up to 1 percent of people. Even home canning has risks. You may have heard tales of botulism, a toxin-induced paralysis, resulting from improper home canning. This rare occurrence results when adequate heating of food before canning does not destroy the poison-producing bacteria *Clostridia botulinum*. A dilemma arises, since too much heating may destroy the nutritional content of food. Freezing is a much more nutrient-friendly way of preserving food from your garden.

Combine industrial agriculture, industrial food processing, and our high-speed society, and what do you get? Fast food, the epitome of our energized lifestyle. It's all about food served *now*—instant gratification. Not surprisingly, the fast-food phenomenon emerged in parallel with the use of automobiles in America. You may be familiar with White Castle hamburgers—"buy them by the bagful." Founded in 1916, it has been acknowledged as one of the first drive-in restaurants in the country. As a boy, I remember their burgers being sold for ten cents each—small, warm, and sweet. I could easily wolf down six of them in a single sitting. A&W Root Beer followed White Castle in 1921, complete with car-door trays and cute carhops on roller skates. A pair of brothers who hailed from Manchester, New Hampshire, conceived the pinnacle of all fast-food restaurants. The first McDonald's was in San Bernardino, California. Ray Crock bought out their concept and went on to found the McDonald's Corporation. The rest is history—the "golden arches" have become an international symbol of American culture.

Sure, fast food is convenient. And when you're hungry, it even smells and tastes pretty good. But is it healthy? The meal is top-heavy with triglycerides, simple carbohydrates, and sodium chloride. In plain talk, it is a blast of high-octane fat, sugar, and salt. Got high GI? Oh yeah! A fast-food meal often tops a thousand calories. Add in a shake and dessert and you're talking up to two thousand. Since you're eating in a hurry, under pressure—possibly behind the wheel—your satiety (fullness) feedback mechanism does not have time to register. Rapid onset of satiety leaves you feeling dull. Bear in mind that a normal, healthy, physically active woman needs around two thousand calories per day to maintain a stable weight, while a healthy, active man may need around three thousand. Where are the green leafy vegetables? Where is the fiber? Where are the antioxidants, vitamins, and healthy omega-3 fatty acids? Frequent visits to fast-food restaurants lead to progressive weight gain. To this, add the decreased physical output of most people, and you have an epidemic of obesity. As the British soldier in the *Bridge on the River Kwai* muttered, "Madness!" Clearly, fast food has negative implications with respect to a person's general health and will significantly worsen the symptoms of knee arthritis.

Eat fast, drink fast, drive fast, live fast—die fast. Slow down! Smell the roses. Savor food with friends. Take some time for conversation between bites. Smell, taste, and enjoy eating healthy cuisine. Break out the fine china and candles. Give a compliment, if it's deserved. Offer a helping hand, even when not asked. Enjoy the dawn and the sunset. Wake up late at night to look at the stars. Take the long way home. You might find it enjoyable—even if you have knee arthritis.

We've traded good healthy food for "convenience" and ease of preparation. Where did we lose our way? We need to return to good health. We need to grow, prepare, and eat nutritious whole food the old-fashioned way. We should enjoy small quantities of it, eaten slowly with friends. Fortunately, there is an alternative to fast food—"slow food." Slow Food is the name of an international movement founded in 1986 by Carlo Petrini, an Italian journalist who saw his country's healthy-eating traditions being encroached upon by fast-food culture. His concept preserves traditional and regional cuisine using locally grown food. I first enjoyed slow food as an explicit approach at a dinner served on the banks of the Merrimack River at Lowell's Boat Shop in Amesbury, Massachusetts. It is a return to dietary sanity, respecting our cultural heritage, land, and people. The result is a delicious healthy meal.

But slow food doesn't have to be "official" or part of a special event for foodies and hipsters. We should strive to make it our normal way of eating. I can't tell you what to eat. The science of nutrition remains confusing, complex, and often contradictory. But I can tell you that we Americans are too fat, and that leads to and worsens knee arthritis. Why are certain diverse groups of people, as we discussed above, so darn healthy and lean? I tend to agree with Michael Pollan that a simple answer is the best answer. These groups eat whole food (or real food, if you prefer) that contains the necessary nutrients. In practice this takes a variety of shapes, as we saw in our survey of traditional diets from around the world.

Despite the presence of fast food and packaged processed food everywhere we look, in most places it is still possible to walk into a grocery store and assemble a healthy meal plan. As a matter of fact, if you limit yourself to the parts of the grocery store where what we are calling "whole foods" can be found, I think you'll find that you will spend considerably less time wandering up and down those endless aisles of seductively labeled packages of food fit for space travel or combat missions.

What is whole food? I think the answer is intuitive and that you don't really need me to tell you. But I will. Whole food is food that has been minimally processed or treated. It is food that has one ingredient—itself. A fresh tomato is a whole food, because it contains a tomato. Ketchup is not a whole food because it contains a tomato that has had its skin torn off (good-bye fiber), its seeds removed (good-bye protein), as well as adding vinegar, high-fructose corn syrup, and a whole array of added flavors, some natural and some not. So you can skip the ketchup aisle and go the produce section. What about meat? Well, why not skip the fish sticks, chicken nuggets, and hot dogs and go for a good old-fashioned hunk of beef, pork, chicken, or fish? The processed meats are full of preservatives and flavor enhancers. I don't know about you, but I prefer to enhance the flavor of my own meat.

The bakery is another section where you should be careful. Look for breads whose first ingredient is whole-grain flour. Those are the best. White flour has had much of its protein and fiber removed from it. Also, bread with many more ingredients than flour, water, salt, and yeast should be regarded with suspicion. The dairy department has lots of good stuff in it, but also lots of bad. Again, a safe rule is to opt for foods that either don't need an ingredients list (because the food itself is the only ingredient) or that have a very short one (that does not contain sugars, syrups, or words that look like they belong in a chemistry textbook). This is the way America used to eat, before we got fat and sick, so let's go back to it. Our grandparents didn't need any special diets to stay thin.

In addition to looking for whole foods, as you wander through the grocery store, you should also be thinking about nutrients and calories. Not too much, just enough. Get to know your foods. Quiz yourself. Make a game of it if you want to. What is the main macronutrient in an apple? Carbohydrate. What else does it contain that's good for me? Fiber, vitamin C, and more. And what about that gallon of milk? "It's got fat in it," you think, remembering the food-pyramid poster you saw somewhere. But you do need some fat to live. "It's the empty calories I need to look out for," you can remind yourself as you heave the milk jug into your cart. Yes, milk is full of protein, calcium, phosphate, magnesium, and vitamins A, B6 and B12, C—and much more. Just don't drink too much in one sitting. You can skip over all those aisles of soda pop, crackers and chips, candy and cans, ice cream, cookies, beer, and microwave dinners. With time, junk food will no longer tempt you. Before you know it, you may even forget the pain-killer aisle, since your knees no longer hurt.

SUPERFOODS

The problem with diets or specific programs for eating is that they are too restricting. From the previous section it should be obvious that with a basic knowledge of nutrition and an ability to differentiate simple or whole foods from complex or processed ones, you can combine foods in any number of ways to create your own healthy and appealing diet. As I said earlier in this book, sometimes the guidance offered by weight-loss programs may be necessary to get you down to your target weight before you can begin using this freelance approach. But there are lots of foods that you almost can't get enough of. They are good for you and often can be combined with other foods in ways that are delicious. They have come to be called "superfoods." Many of them have become very trendy, and a quick Google search will turn up lists of them. Lucky for you, a lot of superfoods may be especially beneficial to arthritis sufferers.

Many spices can be considered superfoods. Although spices have been used for thousands of years in the treatment of disease, only relatively recently has their therapeutic benefit come to the attention of mainstream medicine. Not only does spice flavor food, but it also can be used to control inflammation. Turmeric is a good example. The spice is made from the stock of the *Curcuma longa* plant and is an important ingredient in mustard and curry. Turmeric is also important in the dying industry, where it is prized for its yellow color. This extremely powerful antioxidant has both anti-inflammatory and anti-cancer effects. Curcumin, an active ingredient in turmeric, is classified as a polyphenol—an often naturally occurring organic compound. When combined with black pepper, which contains a substance called piperine, the bioavailability of curcumin is increased by a thousand times. In other words, it becomes much easier for your body to use. Both pepper and turmeric can be added to soups, vegetables, stews, or just sprinkled on fish, chicken, or meat to create an anti-inflammatory delight.

Another very potent spice, ginger, comes from the stem of the *Zingiber officinale* and has been used in Asian medicine for millennia. It is a powerful anti-inflammatory that can be effective in the treatment of knee arthritis. The active ingredient, gingerol, gives ginger its unique, refreshing, and edgy taste. Ginger can be eaten as is or enjoyed as a beverage. Who has not enjoyed a refreshing, ice-cold ginger ale on a hot summer's day? In addition, ginger ale soothes an upset stomach, as you may remember from childhood. Finally, ginger tea can be used as an alternative to black or green tea.

Capsaicin is another wonder-working substance found in chili peppers. This incredible spice is particularly useful in managing symptomatic arthritis of the small joints of the hand, but can also be an effective treatment for knee arthritis. It can be applied as a topical ointment (rubbed on the affected area) or taken with food. But beware! This principle ingredient of pepper sauce is very hot. It can burn your skin or your mouth. Capsaicin also may have anti-cancer effects.

In addition to spices, many fruits have anti-inflammatory effects, including papaya, kiwi, pineapple, and guava. A proteolytic enzyme in pineapple called bromelain has anti-inflammatory effects. An extract of papaya called papain is often used in the treatment of inflammatory conditions. Other substances in papaya include vitamin C, vitamin E, and beta-carotene, which are also potent anti-inflammatory agents. In the vegetable world, onions and leeks contain quercetin, which is an antioxidant with anti-inflammatory properties.

A substance known as resveratrol has also been identified as an anti-inflammatory useful in the treatment of osteoarthritis. This component of grape skins also has anti-tumor and antioxidant effects. Investigators have recently discovered that resveratrol inhibits Cox II, a gene that is important in causing inflammation observed with arthritis. Resveratrol can be taken as a supplement or ingested the old-fashioned way—in a glass of pinot noir with dinner.

Eating a Mediterranean diet is a great way to get a whole bunch of these superfood benefits at once. A diet filled with olive oil, olives, whole grains, fish, fruit, and vegetables is thought by many physicians to decrease the symptoms of arthritis. Olive oil contains oleocanthal. Cherry juice is filled with anthocyanins. Black raspberries and eggplant, like those foods just mentioned, are noted for their inflammatory effects. Vitamin C, found in fresh fruits, particularly oranges and limes, is essential in the formation of cartilage and connective tissue.

Foods containing omega-3 fatty acids are among the most talked-about superfoods. These acids decrease inflammation. Foods high in omega-3s include walnuts, soybeans, flax seeds, pumpkin seeds, and oily fish that live in cold water, such as salmon, mackerel, sardines, and anchovies. Having to remove nuts from their shells slows down your rate of food intake, thus allowing your body to register satiety. They can be used as a substitute for potato or corn chips. Nuts and seeds can be added to salads along with canola oil and balsamic vinegar. Canola oil, with its high smoke point, is a healthy and tasty cooking medium for popcorn. Experiments suggest that fish-oil supplements, another source of omega-3, decrease cartilage degradation.

Finally, green tea is another antioxidant with anti-arthritic properties. Its antioxidant power is attributed to epigallocatechin gallate (EGCG). And last but not least, let's not forget two other powerful antioxidants: coffee and dark chocolate. I've put together a table describing some knee-healthy foods for your consideration.

EIGHT FOODS FOR HEALTHY KNEES		
Food	**Ingredient**	**Effect**
Tea-white/green	EGCG	Anti-inflammatory
Olive oil	Oleocanthol	Anti-inflammatory
Fish oil	Omega-3 FA	Anti-inflammatory
Citrus fruit	Vitamin C	Collagen builder
Orange veg/fruit	Carotene	Anti-inflammatory
Berries	Anthrocyanins	Collagen builder
Spices	Phytonutrients	Anti-inflammatory
Dark chocolate	Polyphenols	Anti-inflammatory

Be aware that there are other foods that worsen arthritic symptoms. These are the opposites of superfoods and should be avoided like the plague. Stay away from sugar, which not only causes inflammation but also leads to weight gain. Read food labels carefully, because sugar has an uncanny way of sneaking into places where you'd least expect it (often under the assumed name of corn syrup). White flour is also off limits. It is converted rapidly in your body to glucose and has virtually no nutrient value. It goes without saying that high-fructose corn syrup and trans-fats will only aggravate knee arthritis. These "foods" not only worsen knee arthritis but also are associated with other diseases, including diabetes and cancer.

CHAPTER 7

MAINTAINING HEALTHY KNEES THROUGH PHYSICAL ACTIVITY

In this final part of the book we have been talking about maintenance. Just as you maintain your car by changing the oil, rotating the wheels, and keeping an eye out for malfunctioning parts, you have to maintain your body in order for it to stay healthy. We have so far considered the ways in which the food you eat contributes to your overall health and, in particular, to the health of your knees. Now I want to look at a second extremely important factor: physical activity. If food is like the fuel you put into your car, physical activity is the equivalent of using the car. Like all machines, cars have to be used if they are going to function properly. Have you ever left your car for a time without driving it? If it's only for a short time, it may just be a matter of a dead battery. But if you don't use it for a long time and then try to use it suddenly, you'll find seized or corroded parts and deflated tires. You'll have to have it towed to the mechanic for major repairs. In the same way, if you don't use your body for physical activity, you'll wind up at the doctor's office or, in some cases, in the operating room.

EXERCISE

If I told you to exercise, you might think of doing fifty jumping jacks followed by twenty-five push-ups. Or maybe you would prefer running around the block or along a country road. Perhaps hitting the gym and lifting weights is more your style. In fact, exercise is all of the above—and much more. Exercising your legs increases their strength and lessens the symptoms of knee arthritis.

I think of exercise and fitness as a three-legged stool. When I was seventeen, I worked on a farm on Wolfe Island, Ontario, bailing hay and milking cows. While milking, farmers favor three-legged stools because they offer more stability on uneven ground than four-legged stools. A good exercise program also has three critical parts and should become the basis of your physical training. The first leg is aerobic exercise. Cardiovascular fitness is often simply called cardio or aerobic fitness. It's a reflection of how healthy our heart and lungs are. When I look at a world-class runner in the Boston Marathon, I generally see a slim athlete with highly developed heart and lungs, with arms and legs designed for running long distance. However, a distance runner's muscles lack the raw strength of power lifter's.

The second part of a good exercise program involves muscle strengthening or weightlifting. Muscle strength is a complex topic. Are we talking about generalized strength? When I think of strength, I think of somebody like Arnold Schwarzenegger, who, at his peak, had developed virtually every muscle group in his body. But strength can also be localized. Think of the arm-wrestling champion who has massively developed biceps, a beer belly, and spindly legs. And when I refer to strength, I am also thinking of power. A power-lifter doing an Olympic-level parallel back squat may do a single lift of over a thousand pounds in a sudden burst of dynamic multi-muscle group contraction. But muscle strength also takes into consideration endurance. Certain activities, such as rowing, require tremendous ongoing strength involving the legs, core, and arms. It should be no surprise that certain high-level rowers can burn thousands of calories per hour. When not on the river, the machine they exercise on is called an Erg—a Greek word that means "work."

The third and final portion of an exercise plan addresses flexibility. The word flexibility is derived from a Latin word that means "to bend." Strength without flexibility would be functionally incomplete in much the same way as an excavator whose arm doesn't bend can't dig a ditch. Strength without the ability to bend is worthless.

Let's take a closer look at these three aspects of a good exercise program: aerobic (or cardiovascular), muscle strengthening, and flexibility.

AEROBIC EXERCISE

Dr. Kenneth Cooper popularized aerobic exercise in his 1968 book *Aerobics*. Dr. Cooper's concept was to perform exercise at approximately 60 to 85 percent of one's maximum heart rate for a moderate amount of time. Exercising in this "aerobic zone" resulted in the strengthening of the cardiovascular system (heart and blood vessels). That's why we refer to this type of exercise as cardio. Fast walking, jogging, cycling, swimming, rowing, punching a speed bag, and jumping rope are all aerobic activities. Generally, to gain maximum effect from aerobics, the exercise should be done for at least twenty minutes three times weekly.

Why is cardio exercise so important? Isn't it just for young athletes and yuppies who want to look good in a swimsuit? No! It's important to start aerobic exercise when we're young and continue into old age. And it's starting young that will enable us to continue into old age. Some of my patients proclaim, "I don't want to live to be old." But I believe what they really mean to say is, "I don't want to be old and feeble." Wouldn't you rather enjoy your golden years being active—with a bounce in your step and a twinkle in your eye, in a position to harvest the wisdom and experience of a lifetime of mental and physical engagement? Living a full life means living life fully. Quite literally, "Use it or lose it."

Doing aerobic exercise strengthens both the lungs and heart. It also improves circulation in both your brain and legs. Better blood flow to the brain means you think more quickly and clearly. Doesn't everybody want to be smarter? And more blood going to your legs means your feet don't get cold at night. (This is why it's important for your spouse to perform aerobics also, so his or her feet won't freeze you out of bed on those frigid January nights.)

Aerobic exercise burns calories too. Remember, the harder you work, the more you get to eat. You may recall that one of my Laws of Eating states that "eating is fun." You lose fat by working out aerobically. You might even lose weight, unless you're also weightlifting; remember that muscle weighs more than fat. Fat, like those annoying little Styrofoam balls that pad fragile objects in cardboard boxes, is 20 percent bulkier than muscle. Thus, although you may not lose weight, all your friends will comment on how trim you look. Then you'll have to figure out how to dress your new lithe and urbane figure.

Cheer up—we've all got problems. Look on the bright side: your knees will ache less. And your doctor will tell you that your total cholesterol has fallen and even add that your good cholesterol (HDL) is higher. Who doesn't like a good doctor's report? In short: fat bad, muscle good.

But there's more. Aerobics transforms you into a red-blooded American. In order to capture all the oxygen required for aerobic exercise from your lungs, more red cells are produced by your bone marrow. And you know this is important because of all of the "blood doping" scandals that have surrounded the Tour de France. More red blood cells means better athletic performance. In addition, you decrease the risk of diabetes. If you are a type-2 diabetic, as your aerobic capacity increases, you may lose weight, and your metabolic condition may stabilize. I've had many patients, who have followed a cardio program, improve to the point where they no longer need medication for control of diabetes. Wouldn't it be nice to avoid the risk of stroke or heart attack? The moral? Lace up your sneakers and get going.

In New England we are blessed with four seasons, and (to quote Ecclesiastes) "to everything there is a season". In northern New England spring begins with "mud season." You'll find Yankees boiling maple sap down into syrup, which they can afford to eat on their pancakes (in characteristically frugal quantities), only because they have just spent six weeks tromping around the sugar bush on their snowshoes, setting and checking maple tree taps. And that's hard work! When the snow is gone, running to catch a fly ball or rounding the bases at the ball field is definitely an aerobic activity. Or have you ever seen our spring runoff? Canoeing and kayaking are exhilarating forms of aerobic exercise for those not faint of heart.

In the summer there's almost too much going on. Walking, jogging, mountain and road biking, hiking, playing ball, Rollerblading, tennis, swimming, rowing, and even heavy-duty gardening (but you've got to dig hard!) will make you feel the burn. And for you romantics, dancing is also an aerobic exercise. Get out on the dance floor and really shake it. You've got to get your pulse up and keep it there.

Autumn is a nice time for a hike. The leaves are bursting with color in the hills and mountains, and the cool breezes keep you from overheating. For the more practical-minded, bucking up and splitting firewood for winter can be

DAVID C. MORLEY JR., MD

an intense form of aerobic exercise. As the old adage says, "Chop your own wood, and it will burn twice." Just make sure you're doing it right—you don't want to strain any muscles or tendons.

Then comes winter. Sitting in the comfort of your La-Z-Boy and watching basketball and hockey on TV is not aerobic exercise—and neither is walking to the fridge for another beer during the commercial breaks. The blessing of snow offers a tremendous opportunity to work our heart and lungs. Shoveling snow can be one of the most aerobic forms of exercise available. Just be careful not to overdo it, or you may risk a heart attack or back strain. Outdoor sports like hockey, skiing (downhill or cross-country), and snowshoeing offer a great workout. And exercise is great treatment for SAD (seasonal affective disorder), a psychiatric illness we see in our northern climes. In general, aerobic exercise can help in diffusing stress in our lives by decreasing anxiety and burning off tension. It's certainly a lot healthier than spending an evening with Old Grand-Dad. And not only does that half-hour walk in the crisp, cold air help us aerobically, but it also exposes us to the sun that increases our vitamin-D level, helping to prevent bone-wasting illnesses like osteopenia and osteoporosis. If you're not one for cold temperatures, indoor winter sports are always available as a way of getting your pulse up, even during blizzards. Playing basketball with friends at the YMCA or Boys and Girls Club is just plain fun. Plus, you get a free aerobic workout. And while you're at the Y, you could do a few laps in the pool. This non-weight-bearing exercise is great for strengthening those muscles around arthritic knees and is an excellent cardio workout. You can even get some exercise at work. Those stairs that you've tried to avoid for years are nothing but a gym in disguise. Use them! Some estimate that you burn eight to ten calories for each story climbed. And what if you're a "gym rat?" Even during a nor'easter you can work out on the treadmill, elliptical, stationary bike, Concept2 rower, VersaClimber, or NordicTrack. Quick sequential dumbbell lifts or a vigorous Nautilus circuit can be aerobic. You've got no excuse now.

MUSCLE STRENGTHENING

Another very important type of exercise in maintaining knee health is weight lifting, or muscle strengthening. Weight lifting should be undertaken as a progressive-resistance exercise program. That is to say, weight should be increased gradually over a period of time, reflecting an increase in strength. Many of you might say, "I don't want to be muscle-bound. I'm happy the way I am." But we're not talking about eye candy. We can't all be like Arnold Schwarzenegger. And then, who has the time, ability, and dedication? We're talking about raw power-functional, "get-'er-done," real-world strength. Remember, your thigh muscles—both your quadriceps and hamstrings—are your knee's shock absorbers. Just like in a new Cadillac, soft suspension equals a cushy ride. Oh yeah . . . (I believe we just had a Barry White moment).

What are the benefits of strength? Many. First, as leg strength increases, the amount of stress across your knees decreases, resulting in less pain. This means that your knee symptoms from arthritis will decrease. Those symptoms include discomfort and pain, swelling, heat, redness, stiffness, catching, giving out, and decreased ability to perform normal activities, such as standing, walking, bending, kneeling, and stair climbing. All these have an impact on both your activities of daily living—like maintaining the household or doing yard work—and your ability to perform at work. I see many patients who present with knee arthritis accompanied by soft, flabby, deconditioned thigh muscles. Doctors call this atrophy—wasting away of the leg muscles. The result is that the knee joints are exposed to all the stresses of weight-bearing activities. We all know what happens when an old pickup truck is overloaded and driven over a street with potholes. The frame is exposed to every jarring bump and will ultimately crack and fail. Your knee joint is similar. Remember our anatomy session? The articular cartilage, like the rubber on a tire, will crack and delaminate. If the thigh strength is not maintained, the knee joint will eventually fail. This is particularly true if a person is overweight.

Second, lifting weights produces weight loss, as fat is burned to fuel the working muscles. A curious thing happens when you lift weights. Not only do you burn calories while you lift, but also the caloric expenditure continues for almost a day and a half following your workout. Some people call this the "afterburn." Unlike cardio exercises, which burn calories only while you are doing them, weight lifting gives the added benefit of a prolonged burn, resulting in further weight loss (passive fat loss occurs as your body recovers and builds more muscle).

So lifting weights results in increased muscle strength (mass and tone), as well as weight loss. Nothing wrong with a twofer! Your body is like a complex house. In this house are many rooms. The attic is for storage and requires very little maintenance heat, since the temperature is kept low in that area of the house. The furnace, however, soaks up a lot of energy because it produces heat. Fat is like the attic, the storage area. Your muscles are like the furnace, producing heat for the rest of the house. When we are inactive, muscle consumes five times the amount of calories per unit mass as compared to metabolically lazy fat. Something else to consider: between the ages of twenty and seventy we lose almost one-third of our muscle mass. Sadly, many seventy-year-olds are burned-out shells of their former selves as a result of muscle wasting and bone loss (osteoporosis). They have bought into society's idea of success—a luxury car, too many labor-saving gimmicks, avoidance of physical activity, smoking, alcohol abuse, the added stress of working all hours. How do we avoid this trap? The answer starts with redefining what is important in life and establishing priorities—one of which includes hitting the weight room.

But the benefits of weight lifting don't stop here. Your balance will improve, as the strength and agility of your legs will have increased. You'll feel younger, your legs will look nicer, and your clothes will fit better. Let's face it: vanity can work for us. You'll fall less too, thus avoiding injury directly.

Weight lifting will strengthen not only your muscles but also your bones, reducing the likelihood that they will break. In orthopedics we often see Wolf's Law at work. This important law simply states that form follows function. It's another way of saying "You are what you eat" or "Practice makes perfect." For example, if we lift weights, our muscles gain strength and bulk. Or if we walk longer distances, our bones become stronger and thicker in response to the added stress placed on them. We are living, dynamic beings; change is the norm. We react to each stress placed on us. Nietzsche said, "What does not kill me makes me stronger." If we challenge ourselves (if the goal is reasonable), we react by improving.

And there's still more! An increase in your knee's range of motion, or flexibility, will also take place. This is particularly important for knee arthritis, as one of the primary changes physicians observe as the disease progresses is loss of motion. Lifting will help you hang on to and even improve your flexibility. You'll be less stiff as you stretch your muscles and tendons. Although it's unlikely that you will ever be Gumby, your knee motion will improve. And all that lifting will translate into overall improved health, including better sleeping, decreased stress, less depression, improved self-image, and greater alertness. You'll be at less risk for diabetes. If you do have type 2 diabetes, you may be able to come off of medication. You will even decrease your risk of developing cancer, particularly if you implement an improved diet along with dietary supplements.

I should be clear at this point that by "weight lifting" I do not necessarily mean "pumping iron," although this can be beneficial. In my mind, weight lifting includes anything that significantly fights gravity. Bench pressing three hundred pounds or performing biceps curls with seventy-five-pound barbells is obviously weight lifting but beyond most people's abilities. However, effective weightlifting also includes push-ups, sit-ups, and wall slides. Your body can be your gym! (Being of Scottish heritage, I'm always looking for a good bargain. If I can get it for free, why would I pay for it?) Later, we'll review a number of effective exercises that improve your leg, arm, and core strength dramatically and can be done without any equipment in the comfort of your own home. Many of these exercises will be very familiar to you.

Now, you may be asking yourself, "Why work on my core and upper body muscles if it's primarily the thigh muscles I need to protect my knees?" First of all, you'd look pretty funny with an Olympic-shaped lower body and a skinny, underdeveloped core, chest, and arms. Also, remember that more muscle mass means more calories burned at rest. Studies have shown that if you work out three to five times per week you can expect to gain approximately five pounds of muscle over a three-month period, even if you're a senior. To maintain this extra muscle, your body will have to burn 250 calories more a day. That means you can eat more. Remember Morley's General Laws of Eating?

Here's the deal: not everyone has as much time as they'd like to invest in these exercise programs. But, if we're like most Americans, when we want something, we want it now. Using the relatively new technique of high-intensity interval training (HITT), we can see quick results with a minimal investment of time. If that isn't a win-win, then I don't know what is. Investing from fifteen to thirty minutes three times weekly can yield gains in strength and endurance. In essence, a series of different exercises is repeated sequentially in what's called a circuit style. Although there are many variations on this theme, a reasonable approach is to perform eight different exercises in sets of ten at a rapid pace. You will be taxed, both from a strength and an aerobic standpoint. Different opposing muscle groups should be alternated.

For example, the quads and hamstrings oppose one another. Do eight quad exercises followed by eight hamstring exercises. Then work your arms. The biceps and triceps oppose one another. So work them. Your abdominal muscles and back oppose one another. They're next. Go! Finally, you could work your butt muscles ("glutes") and their opposites, the hip flexors. Bang, bang, bang! That's what they mean by circuit style. Although you can invent your own lifting program, the wonderful people at Rodale publishing have done all the work. To learn more about effective workouts, track down and read *The Big Book of 15-Minute Workouts.*

FLEXIBILITY

Flexibility is the aspect of an exercise program that, more than any other, leaves you feeling like you've drunk from the Fountain of Youth. Don't we instinctively associate youth with flexibility? And as we age, don't many of us become inflexible—physically, mentally, and emotionally? Well, it's time to loosen up, people!

Flexibility consists of bending. As we've seen above, knee joint motion occurs in an orchestrated fashion dictated by the unique architecture of the three bones that are joined together by connective tissue (tendons, ligaments, and cartilage) and move under the influence of muscle motors. Flexibility incorporates both the ease of bending and range of motion. Stiffness means resistance to angular bending. Saltwater taffy on a cold day is stiff. Michael Jackson doing the moonwalk is loose. Range of motion takes into consideration the maximum excursion from straightening to bending of a joint. A normal knee extends to zero degrees and flexes to around 140 degrees. Optimal knee function includes full pain-free flexibility. Arthritis often results in loss of flexibility, so restoring it is an important goal in the treatment of this condition.

An arthritic joint loses flexibility for many reasons. As we age, we lose elasticity in our muscles, tendons, and joints. Chronic inflammation associated with arthritis may lead to thickening of the synovium and joint capsule, resulting in decreased motion. In addition, following ligamentous injury, scar tissue can form that may limit the normal excursion of a joint. A buildup of fluid in the knee restricts motion. Bleeding in the joint can lead to intra-articular scarring. Trauma may damage the joint's articular surface, disrupting the smooth, almost frictionless, motion of the joint. Fractured bones may result in deformity that alters the normal function of muscles and tendons, resulting in loss of motion. Restoring normal anatomy after serious trauma is a challenge to the orthopedic surgeon but is essential if normal joint motion is ever to be achieved. An effective stretching program is something you can undertake on your own that will help return motion and balance to a joint. Proper posture, breathing, and relaxation are also important in achieving this.

Stretching is literally pulling on something to make it longer. In our case, the knee is bent and straightened in order to restore normal motion. Don't think of a medieval inquisitor stretching someone on the rack. That type of forcible traction rips apart and destroys joints. And ballistic or bouncing-type stretches injure the soft tissue around the knee, resulting in more scar and less motion with time. A knee that's too tight won't bend. Think of a lion waking up in the morning—a forward stretch accompanied by a blissful yawn with its eyes tightly closed. A big yawn and stretch is instinctive and restores normal excursion to multiple joints all at once. You probably do something similar every morning without even thinking about it. You are literally resetting the baseline of joint motion throughout your body. Unfortunately, for most of us, stretching stops there.

Stretching exercises should be done only after a warm-up. It seems intuitive that a warm object will bend easier than a cold one. Try this with a rubber band. Put it in the freezer for a while and then take it out and stretch it. It will break when stretched more than a little bit. But put a rubber band in a cup of warm water and it will stretch easily without breaking. There are essentially two types of warm-up—passive or active. Passive warming would consist of wrapping a warm towel or heating pad around the knee. An active warm-up consists of exercises that get the blood flowing and includes walking, jogging, cycling, or calisthenics. A five- to ten-minute warm-up will raise your body temperature, resulting in less stiffness in the muscles and joints. It also will increase heart rate and blood flow, as well as improving oxygen transfer. If the ambient temperature is on the chilly side, I prefer to warm up in a sweatshirt and sweatpants. If overheated, I strip down to a tank top and shorts. I'd rather be too warm than too cold in preparation for a good stretch.

An effective stretch moves the joint to the limits of motion, causing discomfort but not pain. Pain is a protective mechanism. An injured joint will swell and bleed internally, causing scarring and loss of motion. So take it easy and build up to a stretch progressively. Patience and determination are important in restoring motion.

We've learned that the quadriceps muscles straighten the knee, while the hamstring muscles cause it to bend. It goes without saying that if both muscle groups contract at the same time, the knee cannot bend. In order to get a good stretch, you must relax. Tension, the opposite of relaxation, is the enemy, because when we're tense, our muscles contract. Proper breathing is also essential to effective stretching. Generally, a stretch should be performed during slow exhalation.

A warm room with soft music is just what the doctor ordered to drive off tension. Music is powerful. It affects us emotionally and physically. It soothes and distracts the mind, enabling us to escape to a place without pain. Meditation and daydreaming bring temporary detachment from uncomfortable activities. A trance-like state induced by soothing music can lower blood pressure and heart rate, as well as decrease the production of cortisol, a powerful hormone released in response to stress. Excessive and chronic release of cortisol increases susceptibility to disease. Different people relax in response to different music. Choose what you like best. Singing can be a powerful tool to separate us from an uncomfortable situation. I remember, as a young marine at Parris Island, running for miles with a heavy pack and M-14 rifle, singing along with a platoon of ninety recruits: "Bo Dilly, Bo Dilly, where you been? Around the world and I'm goin' agin . . ." Although some collapsed under the load, most of us continued running and singing with tolerable discomfort, the music having transported us away from our physical reality.

Stretching can be either static or dynamic. A static stretch is done slowly and held. A dynamic, or ballistic, stretch is usually performed quickly with a bouncing motion. I advise my patients to stick to static rather than dynamic stretching, as the stress of dynamic stretching can increase the symptoms of arthritis. A flexibility program takes into consideration several aspects of the stretch: duration, repetition, and intensity. Many therapists recommend holding a stretch for between ten and thirty seconds. Performing stretches in sets of three is optimal. Stretching once or twice a day is good. Again, avoid the zone of pain. A ruptured hamstring will set you back three to six months.

After a good stretch you should feel happy and satisfied, like a smiling lion—purrrrr. Bob and Jean Anderson's book *Stretching* is a go-to guide to consider.

Strength and flexibility improve balance and agility. Both are important to preserving and improving the health of an arthritic knee. Balance can be either static or dynamic. Consider the gymnast posed on a beam, unmoving and not falling. This is static. Or think of tight-rope walker Nik Wallenda, crossing Niagara Falls. That's dynamic. Putting strength, balance, and coordination together gives you agility. Many exercises include parts of all three components. Calisthenics is one example. It involves performing rhythmic exercises at a rapid pace without equipment. These include such activities as jumping jacks, bend-and-thrusts, push-ups, and running in place. Such exercises promote agility, balance, strength, flexibility, and aerobic fitness, all of which promote and maintain knee health.

EXERCISE PROGRAMS

A number of established systems have evolved to integrate aerobic fitness, strengthening, and flexibility. Since these methods will have beneficial effects on arthritic knees, it's worth taking time to review some of the more popular programs so you can choose which one is best for you. You may find one of these programs offered in your area. By joining a group or class, you can take advantage of an existing structure and learn from an instructor. Plus, it's fun to exercise with other people. You get into shape while socializing, thereby reinforcing your commitment to regular workouts. Other people prefer to work by themselves. I tend to be more of a solitary person and enjoy rowing a single scull on the Merrimack River at sunrise. The "quiet burn" of rowing allows me to ponder the events of the previous day and to plan, in the silence of the dawn, the coming one. Also, I enjoy watching other rowers. This allows my solitary and social self to comfortably coexist.

Many established fitness strategies have stood the test of time and have their adherents. The popular ones we will look at are offered in classes at health clubs across the country. Although many traditions exist, I'd like to discuss three that have intrigued me—yoga, tai chi, and Pilates. I've attended classes in some of these disciplines and researched them. I make no claim to be an expert in any of them but am an eager student. What follows is a simplified overview that I hope may whet your appetite to seek more knowledge. All three disciplines will benefit your knees.

YOGA

Yoga is an ancient Hindu discipline that merges physical, mental, and spiritual aspects, leading to "inner peace." The word derives from Sanskrit and means "union." There are many branches and styles of yoga. The popular tradition known as hatha yoga has much to offer in terms of cardiovascular, strength, and flexibility development. Hatha yoga helps practitioners to achieve enlightenment through physical training and is useful for both therapy and the maintenance of good health.

In essence, harmony and balance are sought through focus and breathing. Being more aware of or focused on your body allows you to better assess its needs. Is there excessive pain on performing a certain posture? Are muscles trembling because of fatigue? Being aware of both your static and dynamic posture is fundamental. We are talking about static (or standing) posture when we tell teenagers, "Stand up straight. Don't slouch!" Dynamic (or moving) posture determines whether you glide like a ninja or stomp your way through life like a storm trooper. It is obvious that less heel impact generates less of a shock wave up your leg to your knee. Balance, posture, and focus are intimately integrated with proper breathing. In my office I see many people who have breathing disorders, such as sleep apnea. Shallow breathing poorly oxygenates the blood and can aggravate stress. Deep, conscious breathing expands the terminal airways, producing positive effects. Yoga teaches four phases of breathing: inhalation, holding, exhalation, and holding again. I've tried this and have adopted it into my everyday life. Not only does it help improve my posture, but it also overcomes the fatigue normally encountered around three in the afternoon. Take a yoga class so you can differentiate between chest and belly breathing. Breathing is also carefully matched with specific yoga postures (asanas). A droning vibratory sound can be made during exhalation that produces relaxation—aaohhhmmmmm.

Among the fruits of practicing yoga are mindfulness, self-awareness, and a deliberate lifestyle. Sadly, stress has become a way of life in the twenty-first century. Stress encountered on the road can blossom into unexpected rage.

Other toxic habits escalate stress. We work too hard and sleep too little. Yoga addresses these deficiencies using a physical and spiritual method.

I can recall comfortably sitting cross-legged in grade school without a problem. As I grew older, however, I became accustomed to sitting in a chair. Insidiously, as a result of this Western custom, I progressively lost motion in my ankles, knees, and hips. When I spent time in Africa and the Middle East, it was customary to sit cross-legged on the floor when eating, which I found very difficult to do. I had become inflexible as result of my stiff lifestyle. Yoga is a great antidote to such stiffness. Remember, flexibility is essential for proper knee function.

Since it is a culturally foreign tradition, it may take Westerners more time to successfully understand yoga and achieve its deeper goals. But there's one thing I picked up immediately: yoga improves balance as well as flexibility. I've always had pretty good equilibrium. I'm drawn to slipping-and-sliding sports. I enjoy skiing, snowboarding, and windsurfing. Despite aging, I discovered that my balance is still pretty good. As we become older, we progressively lose our balance. When we're young, balance depends upon several factors, including a structure in our inner ear called the vestibular apparatus. It works like an internal gyroscope, keeping us upright when we're tilted. Moreover, in our youth, nerves and muscles are new and work well. As we get older we depend more on visual cues to maintain balance. If I close my eyes, in my old age I topple over easier than when I was a child. I've learned to keep my eyes open. The practice of yoga helps to preserve or restore the balance of youth.

Yoga teaches that we are like trees. A tree grows up from the ground and is held upright and straight by its roots. This is called grounding and refers to a solid, balanced, and strong stance. It also has parallels in a metaphysical sense that I will not even attempt to explore. A person standing with a wide, low center of gravity supported by strong muscles is grounded and difficult to displace. Balancing postures result in graceful strength. Start with the mountain posture. It's like standing at attention with your feet slightly spread apart. Try standing this way for six breaths with your eyes open and then try six more breaths with your eyes closed. It will improve your balance. I've tried three of the more advanced postures and can actually pull them off some of the time. I like the scorpion because it improves the flexibility of my legs and arms and improves balance. I also like the crane stance, which is like the famous kick in *The Karate Kid*. But my favorite is the tree posture. Obtain a book on yoga postures, or do a Google or Wikipedia search for them. Remind yourself: "This is good for my knees!"

Yoga also works your core muscles. Take away your arms and legs, and you have the core. These are the strongest muscles in your body. They include your abdominal and back muscles but also the large muscles of your shoulder and pelvic girdle. Your core strength not only determines your ability to perform complex athletic movements but also maintains your posture. Try the cat pose, as well as upward- and downward-facing dog. I think you'll enjoy them.

Yoga is forgiving and patient; you can find your own level. But advanced positions can be difficult for the novice. There's no need to tackle advanced postures that may be unattainable and cause injury. A number of yoga positions can be performed comfortably while flat on your back. One such position is called the corpse. As you can imagine, it doesn't take a lot of effort. Or if you feel more energetic, you can do stretches lying on your side, sitting, or standing. Another class of yoga involves dynamic postures. I find the difficult twelve-step sun salutation to be one of the most invigorating series of exercises available. After repeating the sequence three times, I'm left sweating, arms and leg muscles trembling in fatigue, with newfound flexibility. This complex dynamic form is too exhausting to repeat daily. Remember—stretch, breathe, and relax. Your knees will thank you.

Yoga should not be rushed. Meditation is performed softly, deliberately, quietly, and prayerfully. Take time to give thanks, especially for loved ones but also for those who have challenged you. I also like yoga because, philosophically, it is in tune with principles to which I aspire: honesty, generosity, moderation, self-control, gentleness, compassion, patience, modesty, and humility. In life, as in yoga, I have a long way to go before reaching my goal. Just ask my wife.

If you're intrigued by yoga but don't have the time or access to a teaching studio, I would suggest the P90X yoga video for a real challenge. As trainer Tony Horton says, "Do your best, and leave the rest."

TAI CHI

I remember years ago riding on the Columbus Avenue bus in the North Beach section of San Francisco. I saw a group of Chinese seniors in a park, serenely moving as one in a gentle, slow, balanced "dance." As the days passed, I often thought of them performing their delicate choreography in the grass, surrounded by shade trees, rocks, and city walls. Interestingly enough, the park was very near City Lights Bookstore, a famous haunt of Lowell's favorite son, Jack Kerouac.

Tai chi, as I later learned this art was called, is both a physical and mental discipline. Its foundations lie in Chinese martial arts. Far from the study of war, however, tai chi stresses a gentle approach. It is like life; it unfolds in a circular fashion. It is generally about moving in a slow, smooth, and balanced way, like a mountain stream. It pushes and pulls. It stresses a low center of gravity with a wide stance. Like yoga, breathing and posture are important. As with other mind/body disciplines, there is a focus on letting go. It is an exercise in yin and yang, or opposites. Yang movements are characterized as weight-bearing exercises requiring muscle contraction, while yin movements include pushing and pulling, as well as non-weight-bearing movements. Simplicity is stressed throughout the exercise.

As you know, making something look easy often takes thousands of hours of practice, and tai chi is no exception. But it can result in cardio, strength, and flexibility improvements. The forms or exercises are generally repeated three to five times weekly in sessions that typically last from thirty to sixty minutes. Tai chi can be performed alone or with a group. As a gentle discipline, it is well tolerated by many people with knee arthritis.

PILATES

Joseph Pilates was the father of a system of exercises that he called "contrology." Pilates's birth and upbringing uniquely suited him to be the inventor of such a system. He was born in Germany at a time when there was great deal of interest in physical exercise as a prophylactic measure against disease and poor health. His father, who worked as a mechanic, had been a gymnast in his youth, while his mother was a practitioner of the naturopathic lifestyle. At one point, his father established and ran a gym. As a young child, Pilates was afflicted with several illnesses, including asthma, rickets, and rheumatic fever. Being a weak and small child, he was also bullied and in one assault lost his left eye.

As a result of these life circumstances, Pilates became a student and practitioner of exercise and good health. He studied the Greek approach to fitness, based on an integrated development of mind, spirit, and body. But he also studied an Eastern approach to spiritual and physical development that included yoga and the martial arts. Such were the results of his intense program that by the age of fourteen, he was posing for anatomical charts. He became a gymnast, boxer, physical trainer, skier, diver, martial artist, and circus performer. In 1912, prior to World War I, he moved to England, where he worked as a touring circus performer. When the war broke out between England and Germany, he was sent to an internment camp. Eventually, he was imprisoned on the Isle of Man. Being a teacher and nurturer, he developed healing skills as a nurse and physical therapist.

During his internment, he developed a system of exercises that promoted good health that he eventually called "contrology." His system consisted of both mat work and use of a machine apparatus that he constructed from hospital beds and springs. He successfully treated many German prisoners of war afflicted with both mental and physical injuries. He claimed that during the swine flu pandemic, none of his students perished because of the health and vigor conferred upon them by his system. In 1926 Pilates immigrated to the United States, where he set up his studio in New York City.

Contrology, known today simply as Pilates, incorporates proper posture, breathing, flexibility, strength, and balance. Many people regard the method as synonymous with core development. But beyond this, Pilates stresses precise control of body movements, which should be performed in a smooth flow carefully integrated with centering and breathing. It sounds a lot like a Westernized form of yoga and tai chi, doesn't it? And it works too. It will benefit your knees.

FINDING THE RIGHT SYSTEM

After a cursory examination of several exercise methods, they all appear to contain similar elements. Proper breathing, posture, balance, flexibility, strength, and cardio fitness are present. That's why they're all great choices. You can select any system that fits your needs and apply it to you. Your decision should be based on availability of adequate instruction. It's fun to learn in a class setting. It promotes both mental and physical health. Have a good time and make a few friends. Or, if you have no available programs in your area, you can turn to the Internet or purchase DVDs.

Health clubs offer a structured environment with more machinery than you could ever use. You've got free weights, Nautilus, stationary bikes (upright and recumbent), elliptical machines, NordicTrack, VersaClimber, StairMaster, flat-screen TVs, and sweating yuppies in Lycra spandex. I'm old school. If I go to a gym, I like it weathered and full of character—smelling of years of sweat and dirty socks. I guess it takes me back to the 1950s. Go figure.

CREATING YOUR OWN EXERCISE PROGRAM

Since other people carefully structure most of my life as a physician and surgeon, I value the freedom of integrating physical workouts into my lifestyle in a goal-directed way. For example, in the summer I like to row a scull on the Merrimack River. After an hour-and-a-half session at the crack of dawn, I've burned almost a thousand calories. Working out on the water builds core strength, proper posture, breathing, endurance, and balance. Although I'm not particularly competitive, I do enjoy racing a quad rowboat with friends. The joy of groaning and sweating with teammates is an indescribable pleasure tinged with misery. In autumn and winter, I cut, haul, split, and pile six to eight cords of firewood, which heats our house during the cold New England winter. I enjoy snowshoeing, cross-country skiing, and occasional downhill skiing with friends. I walk from the office to the hospital when I can and virtually never use the elevator. I've learned to relish physical work because of the positive mental and physical effects. Some of my most lucid moments occur when I'm doing "backbreaking" work. Also, it keeps my weight down and my legs in shape. And it makes me happy.

Before setting out to design your own exercise program, you should understand an important distinction. Some physical exercises are better for your knees than others. A closed-chain exercise is an exercise where there is compression across the knee joint with constant contact of the leg on the ground. Closed-chain activities include walking, use of the elliptical machine,

StairMaster, NordicTrack, and bicycling. Open-chain exercise involves an impact load occurring across the knee joint, resulting in a shearing stress. This occurs when the link to the ground is broken during physical activity; your feet leave the ground completely during each cycle. As a professor of mine once told me, "It's not the fall that hurts you; it's the sudden stop at the end." Open-chain activities include running, jumping, and Irish step-dancing. Multiple acute shearing/compressive injuries to a knee are not good and may result in cartilage surface damage and deterioration. In short, like many things in life, a moderate amount of compression load applied to the knee is a good thing for healthy maintenance of articular cartilage. However, excessive repetitive compression, especially open-chain, can result in injury and degeneration. Aristotle got it right in his "Doctrine of the Mean" when he advised moderation in all things.

With all the knowledge you've gained, you can begin to design your own program that integrates aerobic exercise, muscle strengthening, and flexibility development. Or you can refer to the infomercials that flood the cable channels. You can watch and work along with Tony Horton on P90X. Many of the ladies—and some of the guys—enjoy Zumba. Dance on! You're getting the benefits of aerobics, dynamic strengthening, and flexibility while having a good time. And if you want a martial-arts workout while contemplating your obnoxious boss, then Tae Bo with Billy Blank may be your cup of tea. Then there's Insanity, which, in my opinion . . . well, is just insane. There are many apps and other Internet resources too that you can use to achieve your cardio, strength, and flexibility goals. BodyRock.tv is not only highly entertaining but a great workout as well. You can use your Google search engine to find a program that fits your needs.

Just keep in mind the severity of your knee symptoms. Many of these programs are designed for young athletes. The key is not to get frustrated. Get psyched by what you can do, not bummed about what you can't. In your case, the old saying "No pain, no gain" does not apply. By pushing through the pain, you may only do more damage. In most cases, it is okay to push up to the point of discomfort, but if you experience pain, you've gone too far.

On a final note, in the chart below I have devised a rough guide to physical training that I am calling the Lowell Plan, in homage the city where I practice. It's meant as an inspiration and a model. You can use it as is, reading back through this chapter for ideas about specific activities, or you can tweak it to your own needs and abilities. You may integrate it with workout sessions and classes at your local health club, or perhaps you feel confident enough to develop a program all your own. Whichever way you go, remember that maintenance is the key to the future health of your knee joints. In chapter eight, we'll look at one final aspect of taking care of your knees.

LOWELL PLAN TO PHYSICAL TRAINING FOR KNEE HEALTH

Monday: weight lifting/calisthenics and stretching (30 minutes)

Tuesday: cardio, including stair climbing, walking, or dancing (30 minutes)

Wednesday: weight lifting and stretching (30 minutes)

Thursday: stretching and calisthenics (30 minutes)

Friday: weight lifting and balance exercises (20 minutes)

Saturday: cardio, including walking, cycling, or skating/skiing, followed by a long stretch (60 minutes)

Sunday: fun day—go for a hike, play with friends, and smile!

CHAPTER 8

ARTHRITIS-FREE KNEES! IT'S A WAY OF LIFE

I've made several observations regarding the aging process. As the years go by, we slow down, we lose muscle, we lose flexibility, and we burn fewer calories. Although there may not be an elixir of youth, we can retard the ravages of time, slowing and occasionally reversing the above processes by altering our behavior. Our bodies are complex and well-built machines. Remember the Douglas DC-3? This marvelous propeller-driven aircraft was introduced in the 1930s, and many of them are still in service. What is their secret? A great design combined with careful maintenance has led to their longevity. As it says in the book of Psalms, we are "fearfully and wonderfully made." With proper care and maintenance, our bodies often will function well for eighty, ninety, or even one hundred years. But improper upkeep leads to premature multisystem failure, including breakdown of our knees. We have seen how diet and exercise can influence this, and in this final chapter, I would like to look at the importance of lifestyle more generally.

In chapter six, I briefly described the diet and lifestyles of several traditional groups of people. Although they were very different from each other in terms of what they ate and how and where they lived, my point was that all of them were healthier than most of us Americans are. I mention this again to illustrate the fact that a healthy lifestyle can take any number of shapes, but all lifestyles that truly can be called healthy have characteristics in common. We can call these characteristics (and there negative counterparts) modifiers.

MODIFIERS OF KNEE ARTHRITIS

Certain factors increase the presence of symptoms of knee arthritis. I call them arthritic stressors. Other factors seem to decrease the symptoms. These are arthritic relaxers. Stressors include smoking, alcohol or drug abuse, muscle weakness, increased weight, bad nutrition, poor dental health, chronic disease and/or poor general health, excessive and repetitive impact loading, trauma, loss of motion and stiffness, depression, anxiety, insomnia, and psychological stress. Relaxers include freedom from substance abuse, adequate nutrition, proper dental care, good general health, ideal weight, good muscle strength, flexibility, and serenity.

Believe it or not, psychological factors bring many patients to my office (even though I'm an orthopedic surgeon). In the musculoskeletal problems that I see, functional overlay is huge. When the doctor opines, "You're going to be okay," it's amazing to see the cloud of apprehension that often passes from a patient's face.

Reducing stress decreases the symptoms of knee arthritis. Lifestyle changes are paramount. Although medications and surgery are valuable tools in the fight against knee arthritis, they are not the first line of defense. Big Pharma tells us we can control knee arthritis using potentially dangerous medication and knee replacements. They preface their ads with, "But first, ask your doctor." Well, here I am. So before you start popping pills and undergoing major surgery, let's take a look at a few arthritic stressors that might be standing in the way of regaining healthy knees.

SLEEP

What's sleep got to do with your knee arthritis? It is well documented that sleeping seven to eight hours a night will increase lifespan, while sleeping too little will cut life short. A good night's sleep enables your body and mind to catch up to all you've done during the day. It is a time of renewal, taking inventory, and organizing the events of the day. There are life-threatening dangers associated with the inability to sleep. Insomnia leads to confusion, mood alterations, depression, irritability, memory loss, tiredness, poor concentration, hypertension, weight gain, and type 2 diabetes. Loss of sleep tends to increase your appetite and decrease your inhibition. This can lead to solitary binge-eating late at night. Progressive sleep deficit can result in a higher incidence of heart disease and accidents. Decreased immune response also accompanies sleep loss and can result in more frequent periods of sickness. Have you noticed more frequent and severe colds that last longer when you're tired? Muscular fatigue often also accompanies loss of sleep and can result in significant worsening of knee arthritis. And when you are tired, things hurt more—including the pain from an arthritic knee. Chronic knee pain can, in turn, result in a sleepless night. Clearly, burning the candle at both ends means the light goes out sooner.

Scientists have organized the sleep cycle into five phases. During phase 1, you drift off to sleep. Your body "slows down." Phase 2 is a light and restful sleep characterized by decreased brain activity. The "deep slow wave" part of sleep starts with phase 3 and finishes with phase 4. It is during this last phase that increased levels of growth hormone are released. Phase 5 is characterized by rapid eye movement (REM) and diffuse body movement. It is thought that during REM sleep, memories are laid down and the brain is rejuvenated. During a full night's sleep, three to four complete sleep cycles may occur. Without adequate sleep, you do not awake refreshed.

As a surgical intern in New York City, I often went two and occasionally three days without sleep. I remember, during one sleep-deprived moment, seeing the pages of a patient's chart move by themselves—a hallucination. Is it any wonder that mistakes are made in this state of consciousness? Sleep deprivation has been used as a form of torture to extract information from prisoners of war. Although perhaps less invasive than water boarding, it is nonetheless effective. Sleep, then, is not something we should deprive ourselves of. Yet we do.

Insomnia has become epidemic in our society; approximately one-third of people suffer from an inability to sleep at night. The cause can be multifactorial. Sleeplessness can occur as a result of medical problems but more often is caused by a combination of anxiety, agitation, anger, or depression. In addition, socially acceptable drugs, such as coffee, tea, or alcohol, can lead to sleeplessness. Our computer-driven society often requires many of us to stay up late at night in front of a monitor. And "relaxing" in front of a widescreen television often cuts into our sleep time. Our great-grandparents generally collapsed into bed at around eight after a physically exhausting day. They had little problem falling asleep. Finally, city noise often causes people to lose precious sleep time. The result of these behaviors can be an exacerbation of knee arthritis.

Many of my patients suffer from sleep apnea. This is a condition in which breathing stops during sleep. After a period of time, circulating blood oxygen decreases to a dangerous level and signals the brain to turn on the breathing switch. A loud gasping/snoring noise occurs. Sleep apnea is usually obstructive and is associated with snoring. But not all people who snore have sleep apnea. It has been my experience that obesity is often accompanied by sleep apnea. The condition results in fragmented and restless sleep. People with sleep apnea wake up tired and drift off throughout the day. The use of a CPAP (continuous positive airway pressure) machine can effectively treat the condition, resulting in a full, satisfying sleep. Just remember, a good sleep can translate to less knee pain.

Not surprisingly, many people use alcohol in an attempt to sleep. But alcohol is known to be a source of insomnia and is associated with a decrease in important rapid eye movement (REM) sleep. Moreover, anyone who has abused alcohol is aware of its dehydrating effects. The restless sleeper awakens bleary-eyed and nauseous, with a dry tongue and headache. Some patients mistakenly use narcotics as treatment for insomnia because of their analgesic/ sedative properties. These medications, however, interfere with the REM phase, resulting in sleep deprivation. If you use alcohol and narcotics together to induce sleep, you may "wake up" dead.

It has been my experience that sleeping pills should be used only for short periods, if at all. Between over-the-counter and prescription sleeping medications, Americans spend more than $5 billion per year. Many of these pills are hypnotics and do not result in sound sleep. They may be associated with risks as well. People have performed antisocial and embarrassing acts without recollection while under their influence. Imagine waking up to find that police had apprehended you while you were driving naked in your car. In my opinion, the risks associated with sleeping pills outweigh the benefits.

So how do you get a good night's sleep? Start by discussing with your physician what the root causes of your insomnia might be. From there, he or she will be able to help you find the right treatment. Your doctor can also rule out medical causes of insomnia, such as endocrine disorders.

In the meantime, I can offer you a few simple tips to getting a good night's sleep. It may be that simply avoiding coffee, tea, and alcohol around bedtime will help you sleep soundly and leave you with an invigorated feeling the next morning. Chronic knee pain can also lead to sleepless nights. Taking an NSAID before bed may allow you to get the rest you need.

Another important consideration is how and when you eat. Remember, most Americans starve all day long and eat big at supper, which leaves them feeling bloated and unable to settle into restful sleep. To sleep well, eat a moderate-sized supper before seven. Don't snack after seven, except perhaps a little protein, like a glass of milk or whole wheat cracker with peanut butter.

Stimulating any of your five senses may also keep you awake. When you go to bed, make sure no light is visible. Make sure no LEDs can be seen (the light on your alarm clock). Room darkening shades can be very effective at keeping light out. Sleep masks may allow you to have sweet dreams. Since your bedroom will be dark, get rid of clutter and potential booby traps that may trip you on the way to the bathroom. Noise can also keep you awake. Blaring TVs, smartphone notifications, loud neighbors, a snoring partner, barking dogs, and honking horns are only a few of the sounds that can prevent a restful sleep. Sometimes the only answer is a set of earplugs. Noise-canceling earphones can also be very effective. Sound and sleep machines produce soothing, hypnotic sounds that drown out distracting, annoying noise, thereby reducing sleep disturbance. The sound comes in many creative forms and includes breaking waves, a distant train complete with occasional whistle, rainfall with faraway thunder, and a singing brook. The "sleep machines" can be set to run for a period of time and then automatically switch off. Touch influences sleep too. Don't wear wool to bed unless you like to itch. Comfortable pj's with soft sheets and a firm pillow may help you sleep better. Get a good mattress that suits your fancy. A cool environment encourages restful sleep. Smell also can prevent sleep. Taking a shower or bath before bedtime is not only relaxing but washes the grime and smell of the day away, giving you a feeling of comfort between clean sheets as you drift off. An odor-removing ozone generator can effectively remove unpleasant smells. Penetrating perfumes or colognes can interfere with sleep. It's best to avoid them when hitting the hay. Taste, finally, can also interfere with sleep. Cigarettes, garlic, and spicy food can keep you awake. It's best to avoid them later in the day if you (or your partner) want to sleep.

Practicing slow, deep breathing, along with auto-hypnotic techniques, can promote rest. Clear your mind. Heavy physical activity within two hours of bedtime can make sleeping difficult. For this reason, lifting and calisthenics should be done earlier in the day.

Getting a good night's sleep, then, is just one more tool used in the multifaceted approach to the treatment of knee arthritis. When you are rested, in the morning you will wake up ready to seize the day. You'll be more apt to eat and exercise better, with an improved outlook on life. Your knee arthritic symptoms may diminish remarkably.

SMOKING

While I have never been a smoker myself, I am not a rabid anti-smoker. But you need to hear the truth. Anyone who still smokes or uses any form of tobacco product needs to stop. It is a scientific fact that smoking is highly addictive and results in disease that affects many organ systems. Since the disease onset occurs many years after tobacco use starts, this eventuality is easily denied.

Why is this expensive and dirty habit so addictive? Tobacco contains nicotine, a potent neurotransmitter. It is, in a manner of speaking, a miracle drug. It "lights up" the brain. Psychological testing of people taking nicotine demonstrates that it actually increases their IQ transiently. In addition, it's has a quick onset of action. After taking a draw on a cigarette, the drug passes from the lungs to the brain in about fifteen seconds. Just watch a smoker the next time he inhales a cigarette after a period of abstinence. You'll see an almost immediate look of profound satisfaction. The smoke acts as a stimulant, giving the user a feeling of both calmness and euphoria. We witness the paradoxical effect of this stimulant when a smoker says, "I need a smoke to settle my nerves." Nicotine is an effective appetite suppressor as well. I see many patients with new onset of symptomatic knee arthritis following smoking cessation, associated by weight gain. The sudden increase in weight can cause asymptomatic knee arthritis to flare.

Although nicotine may not be carcinogenic, it has significant negative cardiovascular effects. The drug increases systemic blood pressure as well as heart rate. It is also a vasoconstrictor. It leads to gum disease and is a major cause of total dental extraction. Taken in excessive quantities, it will lead to nausea and vomiting, seizures, and ultimately death. Another component of tobacco smoke is also very toxic—carbon monoxide (CO). This compound is a deadly gas that binds to the hemoglobin in red cells, preventing oxygen binding. This can result in progressive oxygen starvation and death. A heavy smoker will appear ashen and may undergo progressive deterioration of muscles, tendons, and ligaments. Have you ever noticed the cold, limp handshake of someone addicted to nicotine?

There are many other dangerous compounds in tobacco smoke in addition to nicotine and CO. The residue in smoke is called tar. It is the black stain that remains when smoke is blown through a white handkerchief. Some scientists estimate there are up to four thousand compounds in the smoke—none of them good. You may recognize some of the names: acetaldehyde, acetone, ammonia, benzene, chromium, formaldehyde, lead, and phenol. There are many others, all of which are highly toxic. You'll find them in other products, including solvents, glues, gasoline, paints, and embalming fluid. To make matters even worse, as the toxic smoke enters the lungs and irritates the lining of the respiratory tract, often violent coughing results, which is the body's way of trying to expel the poison. To become addicted to smoking takes years of patience and fortitude, as it is a completely unnatural act associated with discomfort and nausea. If only that same spirit of dedication could be redirected to the choice of a healthy diet or exercise routine.

Furthermore, 90 percent of all lung cancer is smoking-related. In most cases, the cancer is resistant to treatment and results in a protracted and painful death. In addition, smokers invariably develop arteriosclerosis (hardening of the arteries) and coronary artery disease. In more extreme cases, smokers lose hands and feet as a result of vasospasm (Raynaud's disease). And the habit doesn't just affect those doing it; secondhand smoke causes disease in those around you.

Although some people may still regard smoking as glamorous, the long-term effects are anything but. A yellow or gray complexion with crow's feet and wrinkles is inevitable. As physical activity becomes limited because of the systemic effects of smoking, the smoker becomes progressively thinner as muscles and bones waste away. As respiratory disease worsens, the smoker develops emphysema and chronic bronchitis with episodic asthma attacks (COPD—chronic obstructive pulmonary disease). Their lifestyle is characterized by hacking coughs associated with chronic shortness of breath and marked physical limitation. The smoker becomes a shell of his or her former self, living a life of chronic disability because of limited endurance and vulnerability to falls and possible fractures. Ultimately, the habit will lead to a lifestyle of dependency, a wheelchair, and an oxygen tank.

It has been my observation that smoking significantly increases the symptoms of osteoarthritis. The mechanism is multifactorial. Smoking not only directly harms bones and joints; it also increases the perception of pain related to knee arthritis.

So if you learn nothing more from this book, learn this: stop smoking! Use any means available. Google "stop smoking" and read the helpful information available through the American Lung Association.

DRINKING

The use of alcohol is more difficult to deal with than smoking. It's safe to say that although smoking results in a high incidence of disease and death, more misery comes from the abuse of alcohol than any other drug, including cocaine and heroin. Yet the first miracle that Jesus performed, according to the Gospel of John, was turning water into wine at a marriage celebration. The proper use of alcohol can be a blessing. The abuse of alcohol can be a curse. It all boils down to moderation. The problem is that the more alcohol a person drinks, the more immoderation results. There's a saying: "First the man takes the drink. Then the drink takes the drink. Then the drink takes the man." My observation has been that some people can handle alcohol. That is to say, they can stop after one or two drinks. Many others simply cannot stop. Such people should not drink. Sobriety takes discipline since we live in a culture permeated by the casual use of alcohol. There is no question that the social pressure to drink can sometimes be overwhelming. Unadulterated alcohol is a deadly solvent that denatures protein—it melts you! The bartender isn't kidding when he says, "Pick your poison."

Why would I discuss alcohol when talking about knee arthritis? Alcohol is a source of empty calories; you're packing on weight that you don't need or want. It's hard enough to lose weight without eating meaningless food or drink. Also, alcohol is a sedative that robs you of energy and motivation. How many times do people return home after a hard day at work only to have two cocktails to unwind? After drinking, appetite control is lost, and people overeat. Lethargy follows, and exercise goes by the way. This is a classic hat trick: overeating, under-exercising, and disruption of sleep cycles. Some of my patients would cry foul; biochemists tell us that red wine, especially pinot noir, is a good source of resveratrol, a potent antioxidant that I mentioned in the section on diet. Do you seriously think that people drink alcohol as a source of antioxidants? You can get resveratrol by eating red grapes. If you need to drink, do so in moderation. But you're better off not drinking. Your knees and liver will thank you.

STRESS

Chronic stress and anxiety are an occupational hazard of living in the twenty-first century. In the old days, sidewalks were rolled up at five o'clock in the evening. Sunday was a day of rest. Nowadays, we live in a "wired" 24/7 society. Like caffeine-driven Jethro Gibbs says on *NCIS*, "I'll sleep when I die." But there is a price to pay for such a lifestyle—chronic stress.

Stress is not just an emotional problem. People are complex living organisms, not machines. As we noted above, rest is essential for life. Stress causes a cascade of physiological responses that are regulated by powerful hormones. The release of cortisol and epinephrine (adrenaline) affects many body systems, including the sympathetic nervous system. Chronic stress results in fatigue, muscle tension, nausea, shortness of breath, sweating, and a plethora of other symptoms. Chronic stress not only adversely affects your general health but also worsens knee arthritis. This happens for many reasons. People who are chronically stressed have lost control of their lives. They eat (and drink) too much of the wrong food and gain weight. Their sleep patterns are in tatters, and they become chronic insomniacs. They undergo personality changes, becoming, in many cases, raving lunatics in response to even the smallest provocation. They are incapable of regulated exercise and become rapidly deconditioned. In some cases, knee arthritis becomes significantly worse.

One of my doctor friends believes that chronic stress is the greatest health concern of our age. Coping with stress is difficult and ongoing. When your plate is too full, your coping mechanisms are insufficient to deal with the "tyranny of the immediate." Your system rebels as each new, even minor, problem becomes an insurmountable challenge. Emotional and eventually physical breakdown follow. Identifying the root cause of stress is essential in order to treat it effectively. Although pharmaceuticals may ameliorate the symptoms of stress, removing the cause is the cure. Many people are over-medicated. If you have the symptoms of stress, you need to be evaluated by your physician for medical workup to rule out organic or physical causes of your anxiety. A common-sense program, including proper diet, exercise, and avoidance of stimulating drugs such as cigarettes and caffeine, is fundamental. Legitimate worries need to be addressed. Problems can often be solved. Most of us are social beings and need the support of friends during difficult times. A strong social network is beneficial in coping with stress. Meditation may help in achieving relaxation. In my opinion, hobbies are essential. Counseling may be required, and in serious cases mood elevators or antidepressants may be needed. Addressing and minimizing stress is extremely important for the successful treatment of knee arthritis.

DENTAL HEALTH

How does the health of my teeth affect the arthritis in my knee? It appears that unhealthy teeth and gums may aggravate knee arthritis. Plaque buildup can result in both dental cavities and gum disease. Bacteria buildup in and around your teeth results in inflammation. This inflammation can affect other organ systems, including your heart, kidneys, and joints. The exact mechanism is not well understood. We do know, however, that people with joint replacements are at increased risk for deep infection of their artificial joints if they have dental abscesses or if they undergo dental manipulation without prophylactic antibiotics. The infection from the abscess spreads to the bloodstream (bacteremia) and may "seed" to the joint replacement, causing an infection. It is not a stretch of the imagination to think that poor teeth may result in poor knees.

Although there may not exist a direct causal relationship between dental hygiene and knee arthritis, there are many benefits to maintaining proper dental health. Regular brushing, flossing, smoking cessation, and periodic visits to your dentist for evaluation and cleaning are important and may have a beneficial effect on your knee arthritis.

THE MASAI: AN AFRICAN MOMENT

During June 2003, I had the privilege of serving as a missionary orthopedic surgeon in Kenya, approximately forty miles north of Nairobi. I worked at the Kijabe Hospital, which is located 7,500 feet above sea level on the escarpment of the Great Rift Valley. The hospital was in an area of Kenya that bordered on Masailand.

The Masai are a fascinating people. Exquisitely beautiful, as if perfectly sculpted from ebony, they have long, beautifully contoured legs with high waists. Their facial structure appears noble and courageous. Renowned as warriors, they are resilient and deny the effects of pain. They practice adult ritual circumcision. At the age of around twelve, a line of young Masai men stand as the shaman sequentially performs the procedure with a sharpened stone knife. To acknowledge any discomfort, even a twinge or squinting of the eye, brings great shame on the recipient as well as his family. You don't mess with the Masai!

Their denial of pain presented a major obstacle to surgeons. Many of our procedures were done under local or regional anesthesia with lidocaine. Not wanting to cause pain, we could only determine if the patient had adequate anesthesia by observing vital signs (such as blood pressure and pulse) on our monitors. The Masai never complained.

Their lithe and muscular legs enable them to walk great distances quickly. They perform an unusual custom called the jump dance. During this ceremony, which I witnessed while on safari in the Masai Mara, they effortlessly leap high into the air, appearing to float momentarily, before returning to the earth with a graceful landing. A young friend of mine jogged with two young Masai men across the Great Rift Valley floor, covering almost eight miles in a little over an hour. The Masai, carrying their traditional spears, effortlessly walked in bare feet across the 120°F valley floor, dressed in their brightly colored skirts. Their lifestyle is pastoral. They have stubbornly resisted any changes, shunning anything modern and living as their ancestors did thousands of years ago. They have no cars, no Coke, and no fast food—with the exception of running goats. They are exempt from the Kenyan educational system. They subsist primarily as goatherds and cowherds. They rarely eat beef (a man's wealth is measured by the number of cattle he owns) but do eat goat. The goats are grass-fed, both scrawny and tough. The Masai pattern of walking is uniquely smooth and effortless. They stand, leaning on their spears, immobile, sometimes for hours.

One Sunday afternoon I had the honor of being invited to a chief's Sunday dinner. His house was constructed of mud mixed with cow dung. Inside the hut were three rooms, including a central kitchen. The meal was cooked over an open fire by three Masai women, squatted on the kitchen floor around the smoky flame. The interior of the house was dark and filled with thousands of flies. The Masai have a saying: "Where there are no flies, there's no milk." As the guest of honor, I sat on a couch (on each arm of which were six cats) in the dining room—a windowless, smoky room. Dinner consisted of goat meat and a piece of "cornbread." Taking a first bite, I chewed the stringy meat and noticed a crunchy texture—flies.

A major portion of the Masai diet includes a mixture of cow's milk and blood. The blood is drawn through a sharp straw from an artery in the neck without apparent long-term harm to the animal. This low-calorie, high-protein, and low-carbohydrate diet, combined with exercise, has produced people with high strength and low weight. Although I was in Kenya for a month, I did not sample this unique food.

While a significant proportion of the patients I treated at Kajabe Medical Center were Masai, I saw virtually no knee arthritis. Why? Could it be their shoes? No, they don't wear shoes. The answer was optimum diet, low weight, and exercise. Their low weight resulted in minimal stress being placed on knee joints. Their high level of physicality resulted in strong leg muscles acting as shock absorbers and protecting their knee joints from stress. They also had a very low rate of heart disease—an added benefit of their lifestyle. I learned a great deal from the Masai about knee health. There are no health clubs in Masailand. They never attend workout classes—no Richard Simmons or Jane Fonda videos. Their lifestyle is their workout. Our postindustrial, digital society has left us in a sickly vacuum. Time to fill the void. Go for a walk.

AFTERWORD

So there you have it. The treatment of mild to moderate arthritis of the knee is not so difficult, theoretically. Implementing the plan, however, can be daunting and requires knowledge and discipline. Now you have the knowledge. In essence, eat less, eat nutritious food, lose weight, exercise, and get rid of poor health habits. The use of anti-inflammatory agents, whether in forms naturally occurring in food or as medication, can be used as needed. The use of cartilage-healing additives may also be worthwhile. If these basic steps don't provide relief, then evaluation and treatment by a conservative orthopedist is called for. It has been my experience that the great majority of patients will show improvement with a non-operative approach.

As regards the surgical treatment of arthritis, never forget what a professor of mine once wisely said: "The devil you know is better than the one you don't." Some people will require knee replacement eventually, but before you decide on a replacement solution, make sure you have exhausted the conservative management strategies discussed in this book. And remember: there are many risks associated with surgery and no guarantees of a successful outcome.

I'll be frank with you. As I've grown older, it's hard for me to keep the weight off. I have to watch my diet. Once or twice a week I break the rules and eat nachos or indulge in pasta. Although I love a bagel with cream cheese, I rarely partake because of the aftereffects. It's like inflating that inner tube around my waist to thirty-two pounds per square inch. If I'm going for an eight-mile climb up Lafayette Ridge in New Hampshire, I indulge in the bagel—every wonderful bite. I integrate exercise into my busy life. Hey! We're all busy. I use the hospital stairs and park at the far end of the parking lot. I try to get the right amount of sleep. I take supplemental vitamins. In my free time, I like outdoor sports that work the whole body and suck up the calories. Occasionally, I'll visit a health club. I would encourage you to use the advice in this book to create your own balanced, healthy, active lifestyle—enjoy good food with friends while avoiding tobacco and excessive alcohol. You will reap the benefits in years to come. Even if you do develop knee arthritis, you will experience fewer symptoms.

Finally, in our rush to meet physical needs we often overlook the fact that humans are spiritual beings. It took Jesus forty days and nights in the wilderness to refine his relationship with God. He did this with fasting and meditation. It took Moses, Buddha, and Mohammed substantially longer. How many of us take time to consider our spiritual side? In addition to physical health, we need to seek eternal and inner peace. We need to think about right and wrong and practice the Golden Rule. Sometimes we lose our focus: When you're surrounded by alligators, it's difficult to remember that you came to drain the swamp. We all need a daily time of gentle, quiet contemplation or devotions. Put first things first. This will help ease the pain of knee arthritis and may save your life. May you win your battle against knee arthritis.

INDEX

Y

Yoga, 105–107
    benefits of, 105–106
    breathing, 105

Z

Zone diet, 46–47